The Gastric Sleeve

Meal Prep Cookbook

107 Quick And Easy Bariatric Recipes To Make Ahead

MAGGIE PIPER

TABLE OF CONTENTS

INTRODUCTION

The Road To Success

Gastric sleeve surgery is one of the most effective ways of losing weight. It is a type of bariatric surgery that involves altering your stomach and small intestine to absorb and digest small amounts of food. It leads to 60-80 percent excess weight loss and provides an excellent resolution of many obesity-relation health issues such as high blood pressure, type 2 diabetes, sleep apnea and joint pain.

But after this quick and life-saving procedure is the need to the stop the behaviors that led to the obesity in the first place. It is essential to create new habits, and maintain long term changes. In fact, you need a complete change of lifestyle to enjoy long-lasting success.

This isn't as easy as it seem, because it's hard to change a bad habit and build the right one. Changing your diet is the first step. It is essential that you know what you eat and what you can't eat as the weeks progresses. The first 5 weeks is extremely important because eating the wrong foods can worsen your healing stomach. But eating the right foods and in the right amounts will enable your body heal faster.

In the first few weeks, you can only take liquids and small amounts of small foods. Most times only 2 tablespoons of food is all it takes to feel full. Eating solid food is a gradual process that is started within 2 months. Even then, you will feel full very quickly. You may require nutritional supplements as well.

You will continue to lose weight for about a year before stabilizing. You will lose 1/2 or 2/3rd of excess body weight eventually. Consistent monitoring of your food intake by tracking and measuring what you eat also help to sustain weight loss. Have a food journal or use an online diary to do this. You may also count calories. Furthermore, keep in touch with your dietitian or nutritionist.

And you must exercise! Exercise is a vital component of weight loss. Having an exercise plan and sticking with it will activate more excess weight loss. Have a scheduled time for exercise. Join group classes to make it easier for you. Use personal trainers if you can afford it. How fast you lose weight depends on you. Besides, being fit will make you look good and feel good. So establish fitness goals. It is more beneficial than having only scale-based weight loss goals.

Foods To Eat

Stage 1: Clear Liquid Stage

This can last between 3- 5days. The goal is to remain hydrated by sipping 1 ounce fluid over 15 minutes. Take plenty of water, broth and ice chips. Any beverage taken should be non-carbonated, decaffeinated, sugar-free and calorie-free

Stage 2: Full Liquid Stage

This stage is characterized by thin protein- based liquids, including all clear liquid diets from stage 1.The goal is to remain hydrated and prevent constipation by taking at least 3 liters of liquid foods every day. Some of these are blended fruit juice, skimmed milk and unsweetened fruit juice.

Others include protein drinks, light yoghurt, fat-free milk, and reduced fat cream soups.

Stage 3: Pureed Foods

After a week or two of taking liquids, you enter into this stage of pureed foods. These consist of soft foods with no lumps. Pureed foods are usually blended with liquids. The goal of this stage is to eat 60 - 80 grams of food per day and drink 56-65 ounces of liquids per day. These foods include soft scrambled eggs, pureed meats, turkey and pork.

Others include tofu, fat-free cheese, low-fat cottage cheese, strained cream soups, Hummus, mashed potatoes, cooked or mashed vegetables, pureed fruits, mashed chicken, canned tuna, purred lentils and low -fat refried beans. It also includes all the clear and full liquid diets from stage 1and 2.

Stage 4: Soft Foods

These foods are small, tender pieces of food that can be easily chewed. The goal of this stage is to eat 60 - 80 grams of food per day and drink 56-65 ounces of liquids per day. They include ground lean meat, cereal (cooked or dried), rice, flaked fish, eggs, beans, cooked veggies and toast. Here, you can eat 3 to 5 meals daily. Each meals should be about 1/2 cup.

Stage 5: Solid Stage

Enjoy solid meals. Eat different types of foods but ensure they are of smaller portions and are low in fat and sugar. Eat protein-rich foods and high fiber foods. Foods that are high in protein and fiber make you feel fuller longer. Eat whole grains in moderation because it can be very filling.

For about 2 months, eat about 4 to 6 small meals per day. You only require 2 to 4 tablespoons of drink and food immediately after surgery. After a year however, your stomach can expand to take up to 6 tablespoons of food or drink.

Generally, post-operative gastric sleeve diet is a high protein, low carbohydrate and low fat diet. So eat lots of nutritious fruits and vegetables. Eat meats: minced chicken or turkey, baked chicken and fish. Take beans and peas for extra protein. Drink water, unsweetened packaged drinks, decaffeinated coffee, and tea. You'll be fine!

Foods To Avoid

In the first 8 weeks following your gastric bypass surgery, there are certain foods that you need to avoid completely. Your stomach is the size of an egg and eating the wrong foods or foods in larger amounts will cause you a great deal of discomfort.

Generally avoid:

1. Empty Calorie Foods:

These are foods with little or no nutritional value. Sweets, popcorn, rice cakes, chips and pastries fall into this category. Sugar-packed foods and fried foods may lead to a condition known as dumping syndrome, which will make you feel sick.

2. Dry Foods:

Avoid nuts and granola. They make you thirsty and remember that you cannot eat and drink at the same time when on this stage. Additionally, it isn't easy to swallow dry foods such as these. Use low-fat milk to soften your cereals.

3. <u>High-Fat Food</u>

You'll just need to avoid high-fat foods during this time. Food high in fats will make you feel sick and cause dumping. So do away with the sausage, bacon, hard cheeses, butter, and whole milk. Go for the low-fat alternatives instead.

4. <u>High Starchy Foods</u>

Rice, pasta and bread are starchy foods and can be hard to swallow without liquid. They can also cause blockage. Avoid them at this stage.

5. <u>Tough Meats</u>

Avoid tough meats. Chew your foods well, chewing makes it easier to swallow. Eat small bites to that you can chew well. Avoid tough meats like pork chops, steak, ham and hot dog.

6. <u>Alcohol</u>

This needs no explanation.

7. <u>Fibrous Fruits and Vegetables</u>

Fibrous vegetables and fruits are hard to digest. Avoid vegetables like asparagus, corn, celery, cabbage and broccoli in the early days. Over time, you may be able to tolerate these foods.

8. <u>Sugary and Highly Caffeinated Drinks</u>

Avoid sugar, corn syrup. Soda and certain some fruit juices can cause dumping syndrome. Avoid caffeine as well. It causes dehydration.

Avoid At Stage:

1. (Clear Liquids) Caffeine, surgery drinks, carbonated drinks.

2. (Full Liquids) sugary foods, high fat foods, foods with lumps.

3. (Pureed Foods) Starchy foods like bread, pasta and rice. Vegetables like broccoli, celery, leafy greens and asparagus. Fatty foods like oil and butter and also seeds and skins from fruits and vegetables.

4. (Soft Foods) foods hard to digest such as nuts, tough vegetables and steak. Avoid white potatoes.

General Tips For Success

- Eat and drink slowly.
- Chew foods thoroughly.
- Leave a 30 minutes gap between eating and taking liquids.
- Keep meals small.
- Don't snack between meals.
- Reintroduce foods slowly.
- Stop eating when you are satisfied.
- Use a small plate.
- Stay hydrated.
- Sip your drinks; do not use a straw.
- Do not chew gum.
- Eat high protein foods.
- Avoid surgery foods and drinks.
- Avoid alcohol.
- Do not smoke.
- Limits oils and fats.
- Take recommended vitamins and mineral supplements.
- Don't take NSAIDs regularly (aspirin or ibuprofen) unless prescribed by your health care provider.

Gastric Sleeve Diet And Meal Prepping

Meal prepping is a great way of planning your foods to ensure availability and the best minimal meal as quickly as possible. With low portion sizes, the need for meal prep is more apparent. Since you will be taking low portions of food constantly, it is important to prepare meals ahead of time and store leftovers well for future consumption.

Cool foods to room temperature before freezing. Freeze soups, stews, casseroles, meats, soft foods and main meals. Freeze leftovers. Divide the food into single servings. It helps it cool faster. Wrap foods before freezing. It keeps foods longer and taste fresher. It also prevents freezer burn. Handheld foods should be wrapped individually in plastic wrap, before placing in a freezer-safe container or a sealable plastic bag. Refrigerate blended meals and soft foods. Do not freeze veggies with high water content. Zucchini and spaghetti squash, for instance, contain a lot of water and therefore, do not freeze well.

For thawing, place overnight to thaw and then reheat when ready to eat. If unable to wait overnight, thaw in the microwave using the thaw function. If reheating in the microwave, remove plastic wrap and ensure the containers are microwave safe.

Below are a variety of gastric sleeve diet recipes for meal prepping. Some have large servings as they are intended for family meals. Your part is to take only a small portion of these meals, especially when you are still within eight weeks of post-operative surgery. After 8 weeks, you can eat some solid foods with ingredients like honey and sugar. Simply dish out about ½ cup of these foods and stop once you feel full.

Egg Salad

Super simple and tasty!

Prep Time: 5 minutes

Cook Time: 10minutes

Servings: 3

Diet Phase: Pureed & Soft food

Ingredients:

6 eggs

2 tablespoons of mayonnaise

1 teaspoon of Dijon mustard

1 teaspoon of lemon juice

1/4 teaspoon of salt

Kosher salt and pepper to taste

Preparation:

1. Gently place the eggs in a medium saucepan. Pour cold water into the saucepan to cover the eggs by an inch or two. Let it boil for 10 minutes. Remove, cool eggs and peel under cold running water.

2. Place the eggs in a food processor and pulse. Once chopped, add the mayonnaise, the mustard, the salt and pepper and drizzle with lemon juice.

3. ***Make ahead:*** Place in the refrigerator, covered, for up to 3 days.

Nutrition Per Serving: *Calories: 222kcal | Fat: 19g | Net Carbs: 1g | Protein: 13g*

Mayo-Free Lemony Dill Egg Salad

A fresh variation of the simple egg salad to color your morning!

Prep Time: 10minutes

Cook Time: 10minutes

Servings: 3

Diet Phase: Soft food

Ingredients:

2 tablespoons of fresh lemon juice

1 small garlic clove, minced

½ teaspoon kosher salt

½ teaspoon yellow mustard

½ teaspoon dried dill

2 tablespoons of extra virgin olive oil

½ cup celery, finely chopped

2 yellow onion, finely chopped

6 hard-boiled eggs, finely chopped

Preparation:

1. Combine the lemon juice, garlic, the salt, the mustard and dill in a bowl. Whisk in the oil gently until mixture is very smooth. This is the dressing.

2. In a separate bowl, combine the eggs, onion and the celery. Pour in the dressing and stir to mix. Let it sit to absorb dressing for 5 minutes. Taste and add more salt or more dill where necessary.

3. ***Make ahead:*** Place in the refrigerator, covered for up to 5 days.

Nutrition Per Serving: *Calories: 243kcal | Fat: 20g | Carbs: 3g | Protein: 13g| Fiber 0g| Sodium mg| Cholesterol 424mg*

Oven Scrambled Eggs With Turmeric

Turmeric aids digestion on account of its antioxidant and anti- inflammatory properties. Including it in this oven baked recipe will not only improve your health; but provides a wonderfully tasting breakfast of you.

Prep Time: 5 minutes

Cook Time: 15minutes

Servings: 2-3

Diet Phase: Soft food

Ingredients:

4 -5 large eggs

1/4 cup of unsweetened almond milk

¼ teaspoon of turmeric powder

Dash black pepper

Dash kosher salt

Pinch of cumin

Preparation:

1. Preheat oven to 350F.

2. In a bowl, whisk in the eggs, together with the milk, the turmeric and the spices. Transfer mixture to a greased sheet pan. Alternatively, use a casserole dish.

3. Bake in the oven for 10 minutes and when the eggs begins to set, remove from oven and stir the eggs with a wooden spatula, still on the sheet pan. Return to oven.

4. Bake again for 10 minutes or until the eggs are a little soft and set. Remove and stir once more with the wooden spatula.

5. ***Make ahead:*** Place in the refrigerator, covered for up to 4 days.

Nutrition Per Serving: *Calories: 149 kcal | Fat: 9.9g | Carbs: 1.3 g | Protein: 12.8g| Fiber 0.1g| Sodium 192.4mg| Cholesterol 372mg*

British Tea

Prep Time: 1minute

Cook Time: 2minutes

Servings: 1

Diet Phase: Clear Liquid

Ingredients:

1English breakfast tea bag

1 cup boiling water

1teaspoon low-fat milk

Preparation:

1. Add boiling water to the tea in the pot. Cover and leave to brew for 2-3 minutes.

2. Add milk to taste

Nutrition Per Serving: *Calories: 18.4kcal | Fat: 0g | Carbs: 4.5g | Protein: 0.2g| Fiber 0g| Sodium 2.2mg| Cholesterol 0.2mg*

Peanut Butter Oats

Vegan, naturally sweetened and so delicious!

Prep Time: 5 minutes

Cook Time: 15minutes

Servings: 1

Diet Phase: Pureed & Soft food

Ingredients:

1/2 cup of almond milk, unsweetened, plain

3/4 tablespoons of chia seeds

2 tablespoons of peanut butter or almond, natural

1 tablespoon of stevia or organic brown sugar

1/2 cup rolled oats, gluten-free

Preparation:

1. Combine in a small bowl, the non- dairy milk, chia seeds, and the peanut or almond butter, the organic sweetener and stir gently.

2. Add oats, stir and press down to ensure all oats are immersed in almond milk. Place lid on bowl to cover.

3. ***Make ahead:*** Refrigerate for 6-8 hours or overnight. It can keep for up to 2 days, but not freezer-friendly.

4. To eat, open and enjoy or garnish as desired. Or warm in a saucepan and add more liquid, if too thick.

Nutrition Per Serving: *Calories: 452 kcal | Fat: 22g | Carbs: 51.7 g | Protein: 14.6g| Fiber 8.3g| Sodium 229mg| Cholesterol 0mg*

Egg Veggies Muffin Cups

With vegetables like kale, mushrooms, tomatoes and spinach, this egg with cheese muffin will please your palate.

Prep Time: 10minutes

Cook Time: 20minutes

Servings: 3

Diet Phase: Soft & Solid

Ingredients:

3 eggs

2 cups finely chopped vegetables (kale, spinach, tomatoes, onions, red bell peppers, mushrooms) etc.

Crumbled cheese

Salt& pepper

For toppings: Fire roasted salsa, optional

Preparation:

1. Preheat oven to 350F.

2. Whisk the eggs. Place vegetables into greased muffin tins. Pour egg mixture on top, but leave 1/4" from the top.

3. Bake 20 minutes, checking for doneness with a toothpick. Remove and pop out egg cups with a knife.

4. ***Make ahead:*** Keep refrigerated in an airtight container or place each cooled egg muffin cup in a re-sealable bag and freeze for up to 3 months.

5. To reheat, place in the microwave for 40 seconds on until warm. Enjoy!

Nutrition Per Serving: *(w/o add-ons) Calories: 60 kcal | Fat: 4g | Protein: 6g | Sodium 60mg | Cholesterol 175mg*

Pumpkin Muffins

Prep Time: 15 minutes

Cook Time: 20 minutes

Servings: 6 muffins

Diet Phase: Soft & Solid

<u>Ingredients</u>:

Cooking spray

3/4 cup all-purpose flour

1 teaspoon of baking powder

½ teaspoon ground cinnamon

1/8 teaspoon ground nutmeg

1/4 teaspoon ground ginger

Dash ground cloves

1/4 teaspoon salt

3 tablespoons unsalted butter

1 cup organic brown sugar

1 large egg

1 cup pumpkin purée

1/2 teaspoon vanilla extract

<u>Preparation:</u>

1. Preheat the oven to 350°F. Spritz muffin tin with non-stick cooking spray.

2. In a medium bowl, add together the flour, the baking powder, and the cinnamon, nutmeg, ginger, the cloves and salt and mix well.

3. Using an electric hand mixer and a large bowl, cream the butter and sugar until fluffy.

4.Add the eggs, beating well. Add the pumpkin purée as well and the vanilla, beating well. Now add the flour mixture and beat on low speed gently anddo not over-mix.

5. Remove to a muffin pan about ¾ full and bake for 20 minutes. Cool and remove from pan.

6. **Make ahead:** store at room temperature in an airtight container for up to 4 days. Store in the freezer for up to 3 months. Reheat in a toaster oven or oven for 2-3 minutes at a temperature of 300°F.

Nutrition Per Serving: *Calories: 283kcal | Fat: 9.1g | Carbs: 47.4 g | Protein: 3.8g| Fiber 0.8g| Sodium 205mg|*

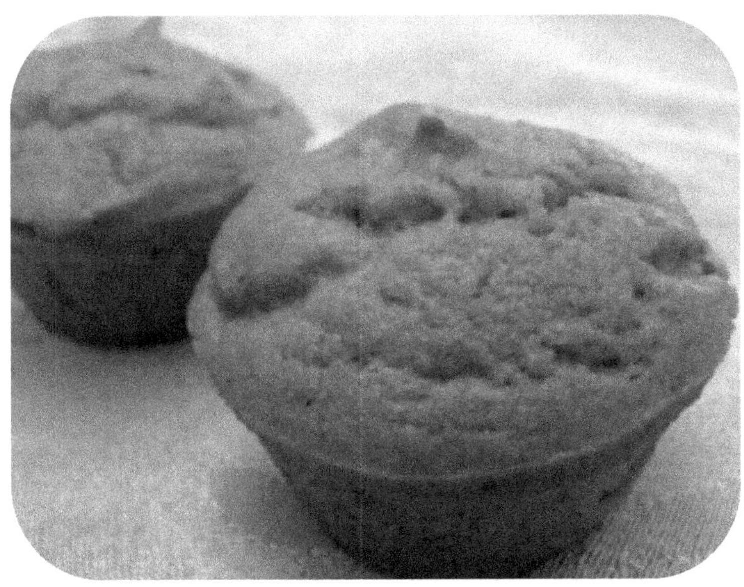

Cherry And Toasted Almond Oats

An easy nourishing meal prep breakfast!

Prep Time: 5minutes

Chill Time: 4 hours

Servings: 2

Diet Phase: Soft & Solid

Ingredients:

1/4 cup of toasted sliced almonds

1/4 cup dried unsweetened tart cherries

1/2 full cup of rolled oats

1/3 cup of plain Greek yogurt

2/3 cup of unsweetened milk

1 tablespoon chia seeds

1/4 teaspoon of almond extract

1/2 teaspoon vanilla extract

Pinch salt

Preparation:

1. Combine all the ingredients in a bowl and transfer in a jar.

2. ***Make ahead:*** Cover with a tight-fitting lid and chill overnight or for at least 4 hours.

Nutrition Per Serving: *Calories: 375kcal | Fat: 12g | Carbs: 52g | Protein: 13g| Fiber 6g| Sodium 128mg| Cholesterol 8mg*

Millet Congee With Pumpkin

Prep Time: 10minutes

Cook Time: 40minutes

Servings: 4

Diet Phase: Pureed food &Soft food

Ingredients:

1/2 cup of millet

2 cups of pumpkin cubes

8 cups of water

Preparation:

1. Wash the millet, place in a large pot.

2. Place the pumpkin cubes in a separate pot and pour water in the pot to cover. Cook to soften the pumpkin for 10 minutes. Afterwards, smash the pumpkins.

3. Transfer the mashed pumpkin to the big pot, cover and let it boil over high heat. Reduce heat and cook for 20 minutes. Stir occasionally.

4. *Make ahead:* Refrigerate until ready to eat and then reheat and serve with a salad.

Nutrition Per Serving: Calories: 109kcal | Fat: 1g | Carbs: 21g | Protein: 36g| Fiber 2g| Sodium 26mg|

Kale & Mushroom Frittata

A simple one-pan meal that can last a week!

Prep Time: 5 minutes

Cook Time: 25minutes

Servings: 4(2 slices per serving)

Diet Phase: Soft food

Ingredients:

1 tablespoon canola oil

1/3 cup yellow onion, chopped

1 cup of mushrooms, sliced

1 cup of baby kale

1 clove garlic, minced

¼ teaspoon sea salt

½ teaspoon ground black pepper

8 large eggs

1/3 cup Parmesan cheese, grated

Preparation:

1. Preheat oven to 350°F. Grease baking dish. Set aside.

2. Sauté onion in oil for 4 minutes. Add the mushrooms and the kale and cook an extra 4 minutes. Add the garlic, pepper and the salt and cook several seconds. Transfer to prepared baking dish.

3. Whisk eggs and cheese, pour over vegetables and bake 20 minutes. Cool and cut into 8 slices.

4. ***Make ahead:*** Refrigerate 4 and freeze the rest.

Nutrition Per Serving: *Calories: 222kcal | Fat: 16g | Carbs: 4g | Protein: 15g| Fiber 0g| Sodium 438mg| Cholesterol 377mg*

Blueberry Muesli

Vegan, gluten-free, fiber-rich and nutritious!

Prep Time: 5minutes

Chill Time: 8 hours

Servings: 2

Diet Phase: Pureed

Ingredients

1 ripe banana, sliced

1 1/2 cups of vanilla almond milk

1 cup of rolled oats

2 tablespoons keto sweetener

1/4 cup pumpkin seeds

1 tablespoon of chia seeds

1/4 cup toasted almond slivers

1/2 cup of fresh blueberries

<u>Preparation:</u>

1. Puree the banana and vanilla almond milk. Pour into a bowl, add the rest of the ingredients and whisk to combine. Place lid on. Chill at least 8 hours.

2. When ready to eat, divide into bowls, add the blueberries on top and drizzle with a little sweetener.

Nutrition Per Serving: *Calories: 568kcal | Fat: 26g | Carbs: 61g | Protein: 29g| Fiber 14g| Sodium 122mg| Cholesterol 0mg*

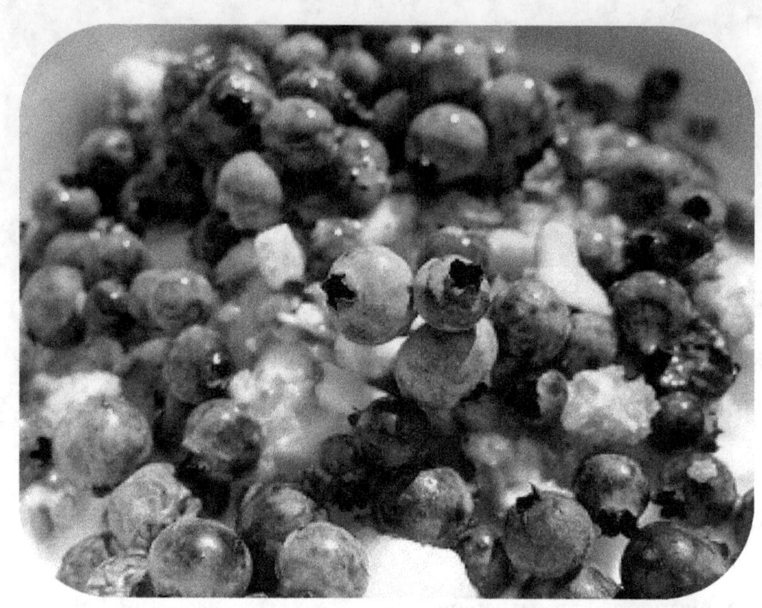

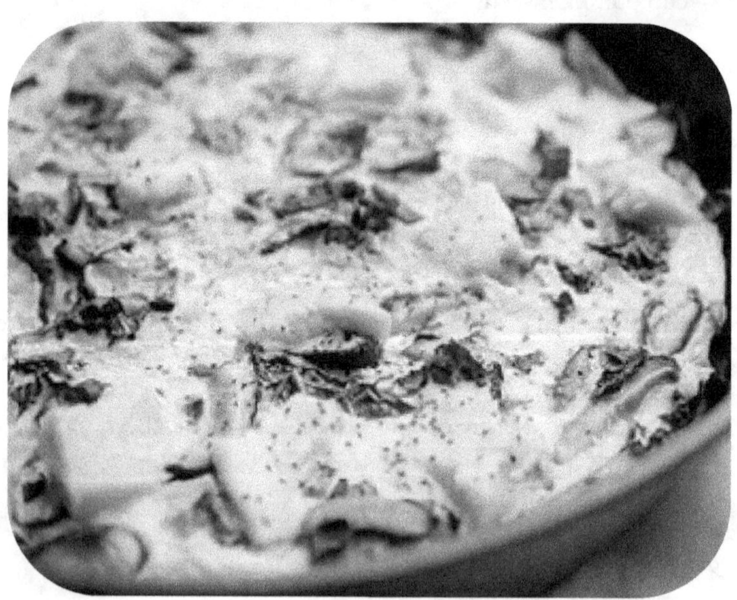

Kale & Mushroom Frittata

Chocolate Overnight Oats

A healthy breakfast that can last for up to week!

Prep Time: 10minutes

Chill Time: 6 hours

Servings: 1

Diet Phase: Soft & Solid

Ingredients:

1/2 cup rolled oats

2/3 cup nonfat milk

1 tablespoon cacao powder

1 tablespoon honey

1 tablespoon of chia seeds

Preparation:

1. Add all ingredients to a glass jar. Mix with a spoon to combine all.

2. ***Make ahead:*** Seal jar and refrigerate overnight or for at least 6 hours. Can last up to 7 days.

3. Eat, if desired, with fresh fruit.

Nutrition Per Serving: *Calories: 329kcal | Fat: 7g | Carbs: 59 g | Protein: 12g| Fiber 8.3g| Sodium 58mg|*

Fresh Ginger Tea

Warming and soothing, this is just what your stomach need at this Diet Phase!

Prep Time: 1minute

Cook Time: 9minutes

Servings: 1

Diet Phase: Clear Liquid Diet

<u>Ingredients</u>:

1 fresh ginger (1 inch) sliced into ¼-inch pieces

1 cup of water

<u>Optional flavorings</u>:

1" piece of fresh turmeric, thinly sliced

1 cinnamon stick,

Sprigs of fresh mint

1 thin round of fresh citrus(lemon or orange), optional

<u>Preparation</u>:

1. In a saucepan, add together the ginger slices, water and any of the flavorings and bring to a boil.

2. Simmer for 5-10 minutes; remove and pour carefully through a strainer into a cup.

3. ***Make ahead:*** cool and refrigerate covered for up to 4 days. Enjoy hot or chilled. Reheat and served with a lemon or orange round.

Oatmeal With Asparagus & Eggs

A quick breakfast requiring no make-ahead!

Prep Time: 3minutes

Cook Time: 10 minutes

Servings: 2

Diet Phase: Stablization

Ingredients

2 cups of cooked oatmeal

1 1/2 cups asparagus, trimmed and cut

1/4 cup of sun dried tomatoes

2 fried eggs

2 tablespoons of organic soy sauce, low sodium

Preparation:

1. Cook the oatmeal as directed on the package.

2. Fry the egg in a skillet until set.

3. Steam the asparagus for 5 minutes until tender.

4. Transfer the cooked oatmeal and steamed asparagus to bowls.

5. Add the dried tomatoes and the soy sauce to it. Top with the fried egg and season with salt and pepper. Enjoy!

__Nutrition Per Serving:__ Calories: 612kcal | Fat: 32g | Carbs: 63g | Protein: 28g| Fiber 11g| Sodium 1121mg| Cholesterol 372mg

Iced English Tea Caramel Latte

Absolutely delicious!

Prep Time: 1minute

Total Time: 8 hours

Servings: 1

Diet Phase: Full Liquid

Ingredients

2 English breakfast tea bags

8 oz. filtered water

1/2 cup of ice

8 oz. milk

1 tablespoon of organic sweetener

Preparation:

1. ***Make ahead:*** Combine the tea and water in a mason jar and refrigerate, covered overnight or for at least 8 hours. Remove tea bags afterwards.

2. Pour the tea through a strainer into a serving glass and add the ice to it. Top with the caramel syrup and then froth.

3. Pour the milk over the tea and ice; hold back the foam and then ladle the foam on the latte.

Breakfast Sandwich

Enjoy after 8 weeks post-op!

Prep Time: 20 minutes

Cook Time: 40 minutes

Servings: 3

Diet Phase: Solid food

Ingredients

Egg mix:

3 large eggs

2 large egg whites

½ tablespoon extra-virgin olive oil

½ small yellow onion, diced

½ cup of chopped broccoli

4 oz. (1/2 of 1 package) sliced mushrooms

1 cup spinach, chopped roughly

1 garlic clove, minced

Pinch teaspoon black pepper

Salt

3 whole wheat English muffins

Preparation:

1. Preheat oven to 375F.Spritz a baking pan (9x13 in) with nonstick cooking spray.

2. In a large bowl, combine the egg whites and egg.

3. Add the oil to a pan and heat over medium heat. Sauté the oil in the hot oil for 5 minutes and then add the broccoli, the mushroom and the spinach. Let it cook for 4 minutes and once tender, add the garlic and cook for some seconds. Add some salt and pepper.

4. Transfer to the eggs and then to the greased baking pan.

5. Place in the oven to cook for 30 minutes. Cut eggs with a cutter into circles.

6. Toast the English muffins and top with the egg circle. Place another English muffin on top.

7. ***Make ahead:***

1. Refrigerate cooked eggs in an airtight container for up to 2 days. When ready to eat, assemble in the morning.

2. Place sandwiches in a freezer bag. It can freeze for up to a month. When ready to eat, remove from foil and place the sandwich on a paper-lined microwave plate.

3. Let it heat for 60 to 90 seconds. It's ready when the egg is thoroughly warmed and cheese melts.

Nutrition Per Serving *(without muffin) Calories: 125 kcal | Fat: 7g | Carbs: 4g | Protein: 10g | Fiber 1g | Sodium 123mg | Cholesterol 186mg*

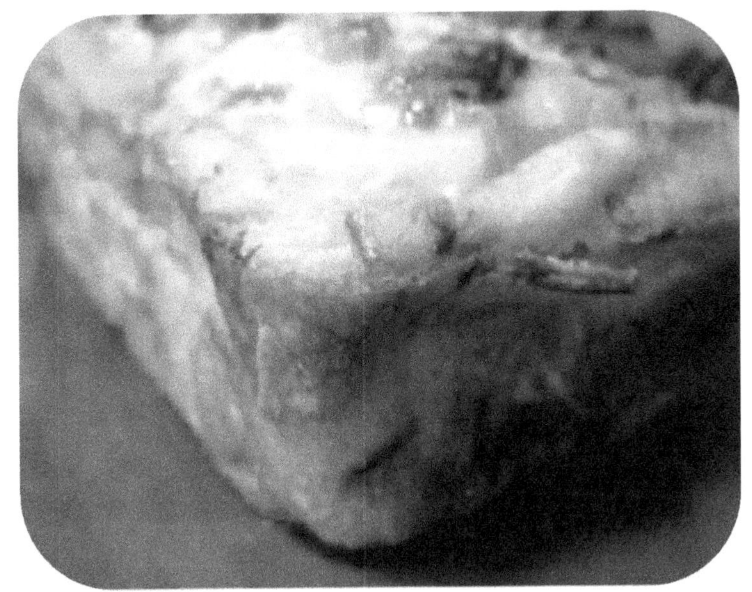

Quiche

Gluten-Free Crustless Quiche

Prep Time: 5 minutes

Cook Time: 15 minutes

Servings: 2

Diet Phase: Soft food

Ingredients

4 eggs

1/3 cup of heavy whipping cream

2/3 cup of cheddar cheese

3.5 oz. cooked shredded chicken breast

1 tablespoon of sun dried tomatoes

1 tablespoon of chopped chives

1 tablespoon of butter

1/4 teaspoon of pepper

1/4 teaspoon of salt

1/4 teaspoon of cayenne pepper

1/4 teaspoon of paprika

Preparation:

1. In a bowl, whisk the eggs, cream, and the seasonings. Add the cheese and then the shredded chicken; add the chives and the tomatoes. Mix all together.

2. Pour into a greased baking dish and place in the oven.

3. Bake at 375F for 15 minutes to cook the quiche all through.

4. *Make ahead:* Cut, refrigerate until ready to eat.

Nutrition Per Serving *Calories: 478kcal | Fat: 39g | Carbs:2g | Protein: 32g| Fiber 1g| Sodium 547mg| Cholesterol 186mg*

Turkey Bacon Burritos

Prep Time: 20minutes

Cook Time: 40 minutes

Servings: 4

Diet Phase: Solid food

Ingredients

4 flour tortillas

1 cup frozen hash-browns

4 turkey bacon slices

½ tablespoon olive oil

1/4 green pepper, diced

1/4 red pepper, diced

1 small red onion, diced

6 eggs

1/4 cup of milk

½ teaspoon of salt

1/8teaspoon of pepper

½ cup of cheddar cheese, shredded

Preparation:

1. Preheat oven to 450F. Line a baking sheet with parchment paper.

2. Bake hashbrown spread out on the baking sheet for 25 minutes, stirring halfway through.

3. In the meantime, cook the turkey bacon for 5 minutes in a skillet. Cool and crumble. Now add oil to the skillet, once hot, add the onions and bell

peppers and cook until softened for about 3 minutes. Take out from heat and set aside.

4. In a large bowl, add together the milk, eggs, salt and pepper and transfer to the pan. Scramble and cook until a little runny and then turn off heat.

5. Place the flour tortillas in a microwave to soften for several seconds.

6. Spread egg, turkey bacon, the hashbrowns, the vegetables and the cheese and then fold.

7. *Make ahead*:

Wrap each of the burrito in plastic wrap and place in a Ziploc freezer bag. Leave for about 30 minutes to cool. Store in the freezer for up to 3 months or refrigerate for up to 5 days. To reheat: remove and microwave for 4 minutes or place in toaster oven and heat for 10 minutes.

Nutrition Per Serving *Calories: 369kcal | Fat: 19g | Carbs: 28g | Protein: 20g| Fiber 2g| Sodium 1017mg| Cholesterol 276mg*

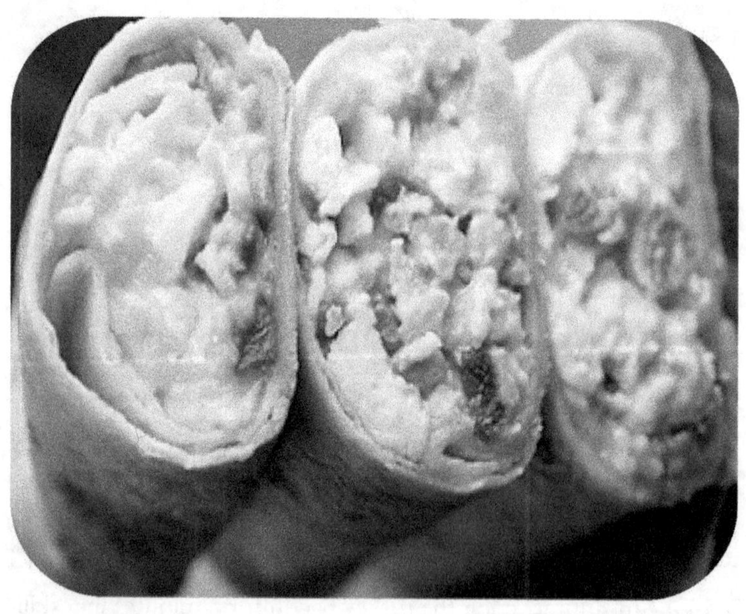

Lemon Balm Tea

Prep Time: 5 minutes

Cook Time 5 minutes

Servings: 4

Diet Phase: Clear Liquid

Ingredients:

1 cup of lemon balm leaves

4 cup of water

Instructions:

1. Chop the lemon leaves roughly.

2. Pour the water into a saucepan and bring it to a boil.

3. Add leaves to the pot, cover and stand for 10 minutes. Strain into 4 cups and refrigerate, covered until ready to drink.

Nutrition Per Serving *Calories: 29kcal | Fat: 1g | Carbs: 7g | Protein: 1g| Fiber 1g| Sodium 16mg|*

Blueberry Protein Muffins

Protein packed, whole grain muffins to love!

Prep Time: 5 minutes

Cook Time: 20 minutes

Servings: 6 muffins

Diet Phase: Solid food

Ingredients

1/3 cup wheat flour

1/3 cup of white flour

1 tablespoon of flour

2/3 cup of protein powder

1/2 teaspoon of baking powder

1/4 teaspoon of salt

1/2 cup of whole milk yogurt

1 egg

1/2 cup of applesauce

1/3 cup sugar

1 teaspoon of vanilla

1 cup blueberries

Preparation:

1. Preheat your oven to 400 degrees.

2. Combine the flours, protein powder, the baking powder and the salt in a large bowl.

3. In a separate bowl, add together the egg, yoghurt, applesauce, the sugar and the vanilla and whisk together.

4. In a small bowl, place the blueberries and add the tablespoon of flour. Fold the blueberries gently into the batter.

5. Transfer to greased or lined muffin tins, but do not fill completely.

6. Bake 20 minutes at 400F. Use a toothpick to check for doneness by inserting into the centre.

7. ***Make ahead***: cool and store tightly in the refrigerator for up to a week or store, covered tightly in the freezer for up to 2 months.

Nutrition Per Serving *Calories: 165kcal | Fat: 2g | Carbs: 26g | Protein: 11g| Fiber 1g| Sodium 117mg| Cholesterol 35mg*

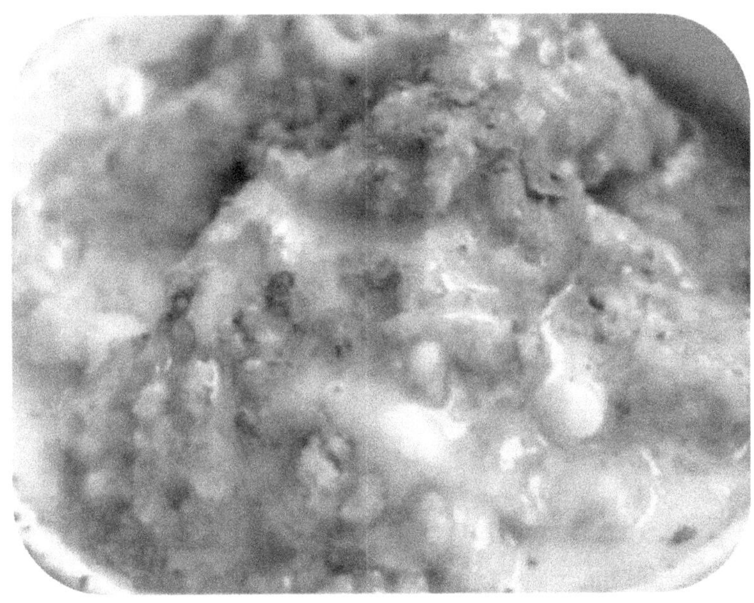

Cinnamon roll oatmeal

Cinnamon Roll Oatmeal In The Slow Cooker

Prep Time: 5 minutes

Cook Time: 4 hours

Servings: 4

Ingredients

2 cups gluten-free oats

2 eggs

3 cups almond milk

1/2 cup of sugar

2 tablespoons of flour or baking mix, gluten-free

1 teaspoon of vanilla

1 teaspoon of cinnamon

Glaze

1 cup of powdered sugar

2 tablespoons of milk

1/4 teaspoon of vanilla extract

Preparation:

1. Add together all the ingredients in a slow cooker. Set it to cook for 4 hours on low.

2. Once it is done, open and transfer the oatmeal from the crockpot to bowls.

3. Add together the glaze ingredients and drizzle to served oatmeal bowls.

Nutrition Per Serving *Calories: 549kcal | Fat: 12g | Carbs: 87g | Protein: 15g| Fiber 5g| Sodium 209mg| Cholesterol 101mg*

Almond Smoothie

A fantastic and easy breakfast made with wholesome ingredients!

Prep Time: 20 minutes

Cook Time: nil

Servings: 1

Diet Phase: Pureed

Ingredients

1 cup of almond milk

1 scoop of protein powder

1 cup frozen berries

1 tablespoon of chia seeds

1 handful spinach

Preparation:

1. Add all the ingredients to a blender and blend

2. Pour into 2 mason jars; do not fill to the top.

3. *Make ahead.* Place in the freezer until ready to eat.

Nutrition Per Serving *Calories: 305 kcal | Fat: 7g | Carbs: 33g | Protein: 31g | Fiber 13g | Sodium 103mg | Cholesterol 5mg*

Sweet Potato And Scrambled Eggs

Prep Time: 5 minutes

Cook Time: 6 minutes

Servings: 4

Diet Phase: Solid foods

Ingredients:

¼ cup of coconut milk

8 eggs

1 large-sized cooked sweet potato, cubed

2 tablespoons of fresh parsley, minced finely

2 tablespoons of ghee or olive oil

1 teaspoon of ground cumin

1 teaspoon of dried oregano

Pepper

Salt

Preparation:

1. In a large skillet, heat the ghee over medium heat.

2. In a large bowl, whisk all the ingredients except the potato. Pour this mixture into the skillet and cook until the eggs are almost done. Stir gently.

3. Add the potato cubes, stir to combine and remove from the heat.

Nutrition Per Serving *Calories: 474kcal | Fat: 40g | Carbs: 4g | Protein: 25g| Fiber 1g| Sodium 117mg| Cholesterol 740mg*

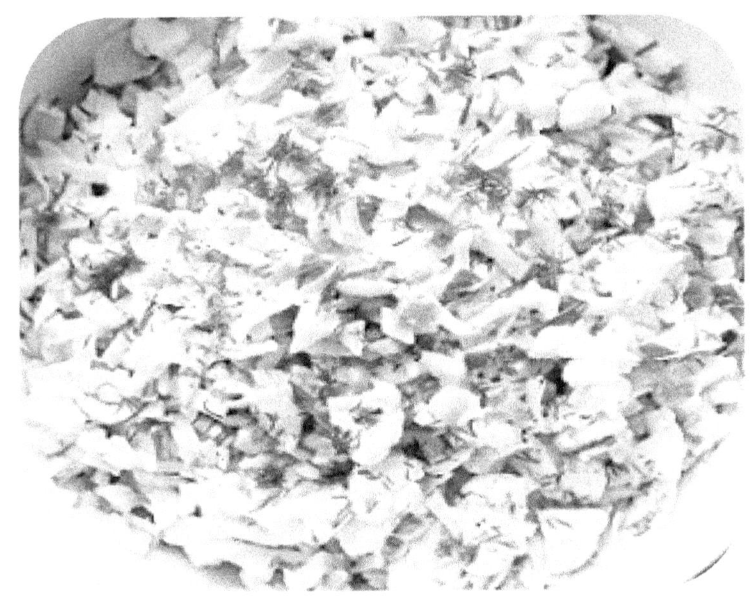

Crab Salad

Prep Time: 10 minutes

Chill Time: 4 hours

Servings: 1

Diet Phase: Soft food

Ingredients:

2 tablespoons mayonnaise

2 tablespoons salad or ranch dressing

½ teaspoon of fresh lemon juice

Pinch of Old Bay seasoning

1/4teaspoon of salt

1 tablespoon diced red bell pepper

1 tablespoon diced green pepper

1 small green onions finely chopped

½ rib celery finely diced

4 oz. jumbo lump crab meat

Preparation:

1. Combine the mayonnaise, dressing, lemon juice, Old bay seasoning and salt in a bowl.

2. Fold the green pepper and the red pepper in, along with the green onion and the celery.

3. Fold the crab meat in gently.

4. ***Make ahead*** Chill, covered in an airtight container for 4 hours. Refrigerate leftovers, covered for up to one week.

Nutrition Per Serving *Calories: 399kcal | Fat: 30g | Carbs: 10g | Protein: 23g| Fiber 1g| Sodium 1364mg| Cholesterol 142mg*

Cheesy Mashed Cauliflower

Prep Time: 5 minutes

Cook Time: 6 minutes

Servings: 4

Diet Phase: Soft food

Ingredients:

1 head cauliflower

Kosher salt

2 tablespoons butter

¼ cup of whole milk

Pepper, to taste

1 cup of white cheddar cheese

Fresh chives, chopped

Preparation:

1. Begin by chopping the cauliflower head into florets.

2. Add water to a medium pot and let it boil. Add a little salt to the boiling water and add the cauliflower florets and let it boil for about 15 minutes until tender.

3. Drain and return cauliflower to pot. Add the butter, along with a little salt, and the milk. Mash content together until it is creamy.

4. Now add a little pepper and the cheese and stir to mix.

5. Enjoy, garnished with chopped fresh chives.

6. ***Make ahead***: Stored, covered air- tightly in the refrigerator for up to 3 days. To reheat: warm over low heat.

Nutrition Per Serving *Calories: 277kcal | Fat: 20g | Carbs: 10g | Protein: 15g| Fiber 3g|*

Greek Yogurt Chicken Salad

The perfect light lunch!

Prep Time: 10 minutes

Cook Time: 6 minutes

Servings: 2

Diet Phase: Soft food

Ingredients

Salad:

1 cup of cooked shredded chicken

¼ cup of chopped celery

2 tablespoons of slivered almonds

¼ cup of grapes halved

2 tablespoons of minced red onion

1 tablespoon of chopped parsley

Dressing:

3 ounces no-fat Greek yogurt

½ tablespoon of lemon juice

1 teaspoon of honey

¼ teaspoon salt and cracked pepper

Preparation:

1. Combine all the salad ingredients in a large bowl.

2. Combine all the dressing ingredients to a small bowl and mix to blend.

3. Pour the dressing on top of the chicken salad and stir well to mix. Serve immediately

4. **Make ahead**: store refrigerated for up to 3 days.

Nutrition Per Serving *Calories: 92kcal | Fat: 4g | Carbs: 11g | Protein: 5g| Fiber 1g| Sodium 316mg| Cholesterol 2mg*

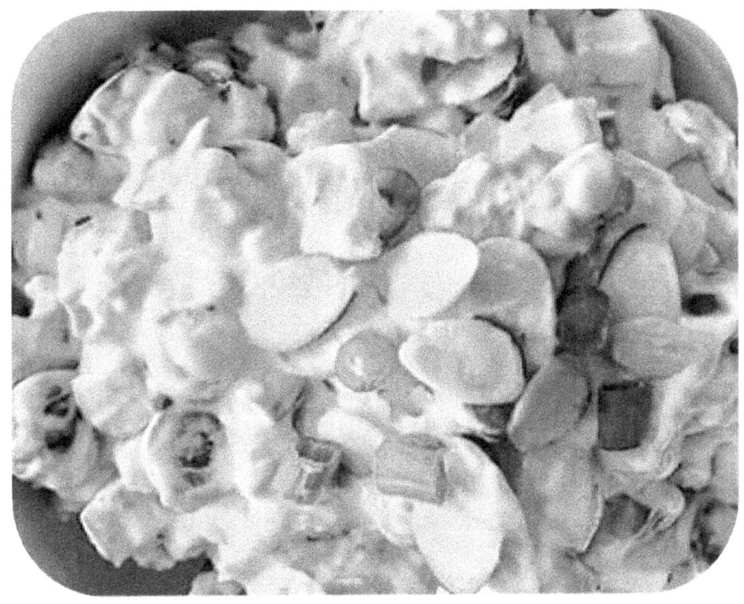

Chickpea Spinach Salad

Prep Time: 7minutes

Cook Time: 0minutes

Servings: 2

Diet Phase: Soft foods

Ingredients

1 can chickpeas

1 handful spinach

1 small handful raisins

3.5 oz. feta cheese

½ tablespoon of lemon juice

3 teaspoons of honey

4 tablespoons of Extra Virgin olive oil

1 teaspoon of cumin

1 pinch salt

½ teaspoon dried cayenne pepper or chili flakes

Preparation:

1. Drain and rinse the chickpeas. Chop the cheese.

2. In a large bowl, add together the chopped cheese, spinach and drained and rinsed chickpeas.

3. In a small bowl, add together the raisins, lemon juice and honey and drizzle over the salad.

Nutrition Per Serving *Calories: 658kcal | Fat: 40g | Carbs: 52g | Protein: 23g | Fiber 9.7g | Sodium 507mg | Cholesterol 23mg*

Tuna Salad

Prep Time: 10minutes

Cook Time: 0minutes

Servings: 4

Diet Phase: Soft foods

Ingredients

2 cans, (10 oz.total) water packed tuna fish

2 tablespoons Dijon mustard

1/2 cup of avocado oil mayonnaise

1/2 cup green onions, sliced thinly

1 cup of celery, finely diced

1/2 cup cranberries, roughly chopped

1/2 teaspoon sea salt

1/4 teaspoon ground black pepper

Assembling:

8 cups baby spinach

1 lemon, cut into 4 wedges

Preparation:

1. Drain the tuna fish, place in a bowl and then add the mustard, mayonnaise, celery, green onions, cranberries, salt, and the black pepper. Mix to blend well.

2. ***Make ahead***: Divide the spinach evenly in 4 containers. Divide the tuna salad evenly. Do not let the tuna salad touch the greens. Add a lemon wedge and seal the container. Place in the refrigerator for up to 4 days.

Nutrition Per Serving *Calories: 396kcal | Fat: 24.8g | Carbs: 21.6g | Protein: 23.5g| Sodium 580.7mg|*

Chicken Cheese Steak Sandwich

Prep Time: 10 minutes

Cook Time: 10minutes

Servings: 2

<u>Ingredients:</u>

2 teaspoons of Extra Virgin olive oil

¾ lb. of thinly sliced boneless & skinless chicken breast

½ teaspoon of ground paprika

1 minced garlic clove

6 oz. sliced thinly mushrooms

1 tablespoon of butter, unsalted

½ large onion, thinly sliced

½ green pepper, sliced thinly

½ teaspoon of freshly ground black pepper

4 oz. provolone cheese, sliced

1 teaspoon of kosher salt

2 sandwich rolls

<u>Preparation:</u>

1. Sauté chicken in hot oil until browned. Set to one side.

2. Melt the butter and then add the onions, mushrooms, and the pepper to it. Let it cook 2-3 minutes.

3. Add the garlic, along with all the seasonings, and then finally, the chicken. Cook for a few minutes.

4. Now add the cheese. Cook, covered for 2 to 3 minutes to melt cheese. Take out from heat and set to one side.

5. ***Make ahead***: refrigerate covered, for up to 3 days until ready to eat.

5. Toast the buns, spread with mayo and fill with cheese steak mixture, enjoy!

Nutrition Per Serving *Calories: 669kcal | Fat: 11g | Carbs: 41g | Protein: 71g| Fiber 3g| | Cholesterol 184mg*

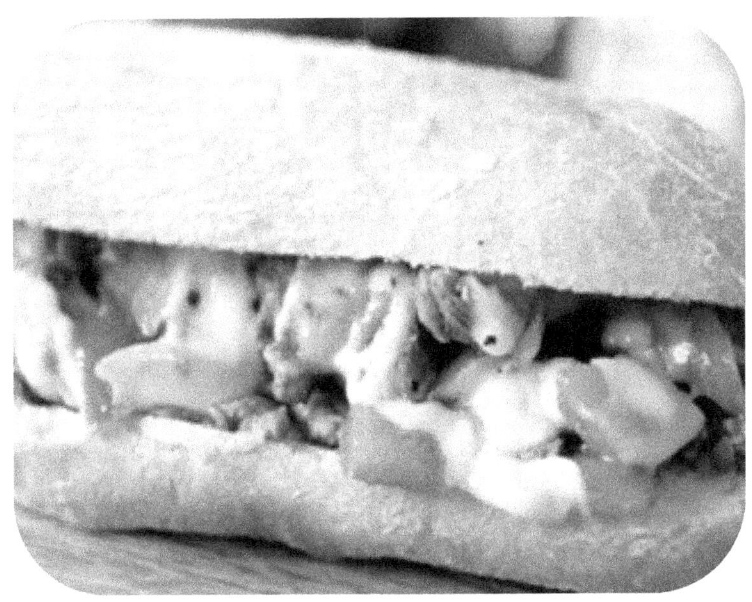

Quinoa Bowls

Delicious and healthy!

Prep Time: 10 minutes

Cook Time: 25 minutes

Servings: 2

Diet Phase: Solid food

<u>Ingredients</u>

<u>Vegetables:</u>

8 oz. asparagus stalks

11/2 cups cauliflower florets

11/2 cups radishes, halved

1 tablespoon olive oil

1/2 tablespoon seasoning

<u>Sauce:</u>

½ tablespoon tahini

2 tablespoons lemon juice

¼ teaspoon garlic powder

½ teaspoon turmeric

¼ teaspoon of pepper flakes

Salt & pepper

<u>Bowls:</u>

Roasted veggies

11/2 cups of cooked quinoa

1 cup arugula

1 avocado

<u>Preparation:</u>

1. Preheat oven to 400F. Spritz baking sheet with cooking spray.

2. Trim off asparagus ends. Add to the baking sheet, as well as the cauliflower and radishes. Drizzle with oil, sprinkle with seasoning of choice and stir.

3. Place in the oven and cook, flipping halfway, until lightly browned. This should take about 25 minutes. Flip halfway through to ensure even cooking.

4. Whisk dressing ingredients together. Thin the sauce with water. Do this gradually until the texture is drizzly.

5. Assemble the bowls and divide ingredients evenly. Refrigerate along with the serve.

6. When ready to eat, top with the sauce and the sliced avocado.

Nutrition Per Serving: *Calories: 396kcal | Fat: 19g | Carbs: 47g | Protein: 12g| Fiber 13g| Sodium 80mg| Cholesterol 8mg*

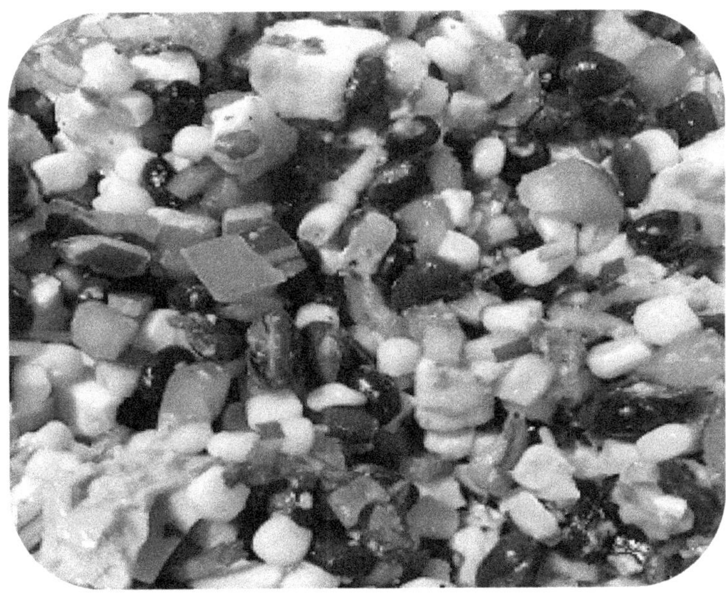

Black Bean Salsa

Black Bean Salsa

Prep/Total Time: 20 minutes

Servings: 3-1/2 cups

Diet Phase: Soft food

Ingredients:

1 15- ounce can black beans, rinsed and drained

1 medium cucumber, seeded chopped

½ cup of chopped tomato

½ cup of green onions, sliced

¼ cup of lime juice

1 tablespoon of snipped fresh cilantro

1 tablespoon of olive oil

½ teaspoon ground cumin

1/3 teaspoon salt

1/3 teaspoon cayenne pepper

Preparation:

1. Add together all the ingredients in a bowl, cover and refrigerate for 4 hours.

2. Enjoy over grilled meat.

3. *Make ahead*: refrigerate, covered, for up to 24 hours.

Nutrition Per Serving Calories: 35kcal | Fat: 1g | Carbs: 6g | Protein: 2g| Fiber 2g| 98 mg sodium | Cholesterol 0mg

Caesar Salad

Prep Time: 10 minutes

Cook Time: 10 minutes

Servings: 3

Diet Phase: Solid food

<u>Ingredients:</u>

Croutons:

½ tablespoon olive oil

¾ - 1 cup bread cubes (a day-old)

1/4 teaspoon of kosher salt

Dressing:

¼ (2 oz.) can anchovy fillets, oil-packed, drained

1 small cloves garlic, chopped coarsely

1 large egg yolk

1/4 teaspoon Dijon mustard

1/2 tablespoon fresh lemon juice

½ tablespoon olive oil

2 tablespoons of vegetable oil

1 tablespoon Parmesan cheese, finely grated

Freshly ground black pepper

Salad:

3/4 medium hearts romaine lettuce

1 oz. Parmesan cheese, shaved with a vegetable peeler

Preparation:

1. Add oil to pan and heat and once hot, add the bread cubes, sprinkle with salt and stir to coat with the oil. Toast and toss the bread cubes for 5 minutes until golden brown. Remove and let it cool.

2. Mix the garlic and anchovies together until paste-like.

3. Whisk the egg yolk in a bowl. Add the mustard and whisk. Add the anchovy-garlic mixture. Whisk. Add the lemon juice and whisk to mix all.

4. Now add the olive oil and whisk to thicken for a minute or less. Pour in the vegetable oil and add the cheese. Season with black pepper.

5. Cut the romaine into pieces, rinse and pat dry.

6. Place the romaine in a bowl, add ½ of the dressing and mix.Add the croutons, toss and add some more cheese and pepper as needed.

7. *Make ahead:*

Make croutons 3 days ahead and store at room temperature in an airtight container for up to 1 week.

Store in the freezer for up to 6 months. Store the leftover dressing in the refrigerator for up to a week.

Nutrition Per Serving *Calories: 591kcal | Fat: 43g | Carbs: 15g | Protein: 30g| Fiber 2g| 2130mg sodium| Cholesterol 148mg*

Baked Chicken Pesto

Prep Time: 10 minutes

Cook Time: 30 minutes

Servings: 2

Diet Phase: Solid food

Ingredients:

2 teaspoons of basil pesto

1 small tomatoes, thinly sliced

1 lb. chicken breasts, boneless & skinless

3 tablespoons of mozzarella cheese, shredded

1 teaspoon of parmesan cheese, grated

Kosher salt and fresh pepper to taste

Preparation:

1. Preheat your oven to 400F; next line a large baking sheet with foil.

2. Make 2 very thin cutlets of chicken by slicing it horizontally, place the chicken in a large bowl and sprinkle with salt and pepper to season.

3. Place chicken on the foil-lined baking sheet, arrange well and spoon a teaspoon of pesto over each chicken piece. Bake for 25 minutes in the oven.

4. Remove, top with tomatoes and cheeses. Return to the oven to melt cheese.

Nutrition Per Serving *Calories: 205kcal | Fat: 11g | Carbs: 2.5g | Protein: 30g | Fiber 0.5g | Sodium: 171.5mg | Cholesterol 90.5mg*

Couscous Salad with Basil & Tomatoes

Prep Time: 15 minutes

Cook Time: 10 minutes

Servings: 3

Diet Phase: Solid food

Ingredients:

¼ teaspoon of salt

¾ cup of couscous

2 tablespoon of crumbled feta cheese

¾ tablespoon of olive oil

1clove of minced garlic

7 oz. chicken broth

1 cup of fresh chopped tomato

2 tablespoons of basil, thinly sliced

1 tablespoons of balsamic vinegar

Pinch ground black pepper

½ tablespoon of extra-virgin olive oil

Preparation:

1. Heat the olive oil add garlic to it and cook a few minutes.

2. Pour in the chicken broth and let it cook for 5 minutes; add the couscous to the simmering dish, cover and cook 5 minutes to absorb liquid. Remove from heat

3. Stir in the chopped tomatoes, the vinegar along with the rest of the ingredients, stir to mix.

Nutrition Per Serving *Calories: 142kcal | Fat: 7g | Carbs: 14g | Protein: 6g| Fiber 2g|Sodium: 263mg | Cholesterol 7mg*

Baked Veggie Frittata

Prep Time: 10 minutes

Cook Time: 20 minutes

Serving: 2

Ingredients:

3 eggs

1/3 cup of chopped spinach

2 spring onions, finely chopped

11/2 tablespoons of soft cheese

Soft flatbreads to serve

1 tablespoon of olive oil

1/3 cups of cheddar, finely grated(half of 1/3 cup?)

1 roasted red pepper, diced

A medium handful of coriander, chopped

1 tablespoon of sliced pickled jalapeños, drained and chopped

Preparation:

1. Preheat your oven to 356F and line a deep flan tin with foil.

2. Add olive oil in a saucepan and heat; sauté onions in it until tender. Add the spinach now and cook until wilted. Season and let it cool.

3. Place the cheese in a bowl; add the eggs and the seasoning and whisk to mix.

4. Stir in the spinach, the jalapeños, the cheddar, coriander and pepper. Mix and remove to baking sheet. Let it bake for 10 minutes until set.

5. Remove and set cool before serving with flatbread, enjoy!

Nutrition Per Serving*Calories: 454kcal | Fat: 34g | Carbs: 17g | Protein: 21g| Fiber 2g|Sodium: 1142mg | Cholesterol 339mg*

Cucumber Tomato Salad

Prep/Total Time: 20minutes

Servings: 2

Diet Phase: Solid foods

Ingredients

1 medium English cucumber sliced

2 medium tomatoes diced

¼ red onion sliced

½ tablespoon fresh parsley

1 tablespoons olive oil

½ tablespoon red wine vinegar

Salt& pepper to taste

Preparation:

1. Combine all the ingredients in a bowl. Toss thoroughly to mix.

2. Chill for at least 20 minutes before eating

3. ***Make ahead***: whisk the wine vinegar, oil, parsley, salt and pepper in the salad bowl. Peel onion, cut into slivers and add to the vinaigrette. This enables the flavor to blend. Refrigerate, covered for a whole day. To assemble salad, simply slice the tomatoes and cucumber and add to the onion and vinaigrette mixture. Chill for 30 minutes before serving.

Nutrition Per Serving *Calories: 104kcal | Fat: 8g | Carbs: 7g | Protein: 2g| Fiber 2g| Sodium: 6mg |*

Crab Stuffed Avocado

Prep/Total Time: 10minutes

Servings: 4

Diet Phase: Soft foods

<u>Ingredients</u>

12 oz. lump crab meat

1/3 cup Greek yogurt

1/2 red onion, minced

2 tablespoons chives, chopped

3 tablespoons lemon juice

Kosher salt

1/2 teaspoon cayenne pepper

1 cup cheddar, shredded

2 avocados, halved & pitted

<u>Preparation:</u>

1. Combine the crab meat, the Greek yoghurt, onion, chives, juice of lemon and the cayenne in a bowl. Sprinkle with a little salt.

2. Scoop out the avocados but leave a small border. Dice the avocado flesh and add to the crab mixture, folding in.

3. Preheat your broiler. Place the crab mixture to the avocado bowls and add cheddar on top. Place in the broiler and cook for a minute to melt cheese.

4. Serve immediately!

Nutrition Per Serving *Calories: 350kcal | Fat: 21g | Carbs: 9g | Protein: 30g| Fiber 5g|Sodium: 510mg |*

Meat Loaf

Prep Time: 20 minutes

Total Time: 60 minutes

Servings: 2

Diet Phase: Solid food

Ingredients

10- 12 oz. lean ground beef

½ cup milk

½ tablespoon of Worcestershire Sauce

½ teaspoon of fresh sage leaves, chopped

½ teaspoon of salt

¼ teaspoon of pepper

¼ teaspoon of ground mustard

1 garlic clove, chopped

¼ cup of bread crumbs

1 small egg

1 small onion, diced

Preparation:

1. Add all ingredients together.

2. Form into a loaf and place in ungreased pan.

3. Bake in the oven at 350° for 1 hour. Do not cover. Remove when an inserted thermometer reads 160°F

4. ***Make ahead***: Wrap the pan in saran and then cover with foil. Date it and place in the freezer for up to 6 months. When ready to eat, preheat oven to 350°F.Bakefor 1 hour. Do not cover. Remove when an inserted thermometer reads 160°F. Cool and serve.

Quick Fish Curry

Prep Time: 5minutes

Total Time: 25minutes

Servings: 4

Diet Phase: Soft food

Ingredients

2 tablespoons of extra virgin olive oil

1 small yellow onion, chopped finely

2 tablespoons of grated ginger

2 cloves garlic, minced

1 tablespoon of curry powder

1 cup of coconut cream

1 cup stock or water

2 medium tomatoes, chopped

4 thick skinless fillets, cut into ½ inches

Preparation:

1. Add oil to a pan and heat and then add the onion, cooking and stirring for about 5 minutes until just brown.

2. Add the tomatoes, ginger and garlic and let it cook for a minute. Add the curry powder and let it cook for a minute longer.

3. Add the coconut cream gently and pour in the stock, let it simmer and cook for 7 minutes.

4. Add the fish and gently cook through for 6-8minutes

5, divide and serve, topped as desired.

6. ***Make ahead***: make the sauce and transfer to an airtight container. Refrigerate for up to 3 days. When ready to eat, bring the sauce to a simmer and now add the fish. Let it cook through.

Nutrition Per Serving *Calories: 431kcal | Fat: 31.6g | Carbs: 9.3g | Protein: 30.1g| Fiber 3.1g|Sodium: 168mg |*

Italian Chicken Puree

Prep/Total Time: 5minutes

Servings: 1

Diet Phase: Pureed diet

Ingredients

1/4 cup of canned chicken

1 1/2 tablespoon of tomato sauce

1/8 teaspoon of sea salt

1/8 teaspoon of fresh ground pepper

1 teaspoon of Italian seasoning

Preparation:

1. Puree all ingredients in a blender until softened.

2. Alternatively, blend all ingredients with the back of a spoon until thoroughly incorporated.

Nutrition Per Serving *Calories: 88kcal | Fat: 2g | Carbs: 5g | Protein: 14g| Fiber 1g|Sodium: 667mg | Cholesterol 45mg*

Mac And Cheese

Enjoy with family and friends anytime of the day!

Prep Time: 10 minutes

Total Time: 15minutes

Servings: 6

Diet Phase: Soft food

Ingredients

¾ pound short pasta

2 tablespoons of butter

¼ cup flour

4 cups whole milk

8 oz. (about 2 cups) shredded Cheddar-Jack cheese

½ teaspoon black pepper

1 tablespoon Dijon mustard

5 slices (about 4 oz.)Muenster cheese

Preparation:

1. Cook the pasta as directed on the package.

2. Melt the butter in a pot. Add the flour. Cook and stir for 2 minutes and then add the milk gently. Stir and cook for about 8 minutes until the sauce is a little thick.

3. Now add the cheddar cheese, the mustard, and pepper and let it melt. Add the pasta and stir.

4. Remove to a baking dish, Top with the Muenster cheese.

5. ***Make ahead***: cover with a plastic wrap tightly and refrigerate for up to 4 days. When ready to eat, bring to room temperature and Bake for 35 minutes at 400° F until golden.

Nutrition Per Serving *Calories: 550kcal | Fat: 24g | Carbs: 56g | Protein: 26g| Fiber 2g|Sodium: 480mg | Cholesterol 70mg*

Spicy Buffalo Chicken Wraps

Prep/Total Time: 5minutes

Servings: 4

Diet Phase: Soft food

Ingredients

2 cup of cooked shredded chicken

1/2 cup buffalo sauce

1 cup of shredded lettuce

1/4 cup ranch dressing

4 medium flour tortillas

Preparation:

1. Coat the cooked chicken in the buffalo sauce.

2. Lay flour tortilla out and divide mixture among the tortillas evenly. Add the lettuce and ranch dressing to top and then fold the tortilla sides and roll up.

3. Eat warm or cold.

4. ***Make ahead***: Prepare individual ingredients and store in the refrigerator for up to 3 days. When ready to eat, assemble. Do not store leftovers.

Nutrition Per Serving *Calories: 263kcal | Fat: 12g | Carbs: 16g | Protein: 20g| Fiber0|Sodium: 1321mg | Cholesterol 53mg*

Spicy Thai Shrimp Lettuce Wraps With Peanut Sauce

Prep/Total Time: 15minutes

Servings: 4

Diet Phase: Soft food

Ingredients

Thai Shrimp:

1 lb. shrimp (peeled &de-veined)

2 tablespoons of coconut aminos

1/4 cup olive oil

1 tablespoon of fish sauce

1/4 teaspoon of crushed red pepper flakes

2 teaspoon of lime juice

 Lettuce wraps:

16 leaves bibb lettuce

1 large avocado, diced

1/3 small cucumber (3 oz. julienned)

Peanut Sauce:

1/4 cup peanut butter

1/4 cup coconut aminos

1/2 teaspoon of crushed red pepper flakes

1 1/2 tablespoon of lime juice

1/4teaspoon of sea salt

<u>**Preparation:**</u>

1. Cover the coconut aminos, 2 tablespoons of oil, the fish sauce, crushed red pepper and lime juice in a bowl

2. Add the shrimp and toss to coat. Place lid on and leave to marinate for 30 minutes.

3. Next, combine the peanut sauce ingredients together and set to one side.

4. Add the rest of the oil to a pan and heat. Sauté the shrimp in the oil for 5 minutes until opaque.

5. Lay out lettuce leaves and place the shrimp, the cucumbers and the avocados on it, dividing evenly. Drizzle with the peanut sauce. Garnish as desired.

6. ***Make ahead:*** pack properly and store in the refrigerator for up to 3 days.

Nutrition Per Serving *Calories: 470kcal | Fat: 31g | Carbs: 16g | Protein: 29g| Fiber6| Net Carbs10g*

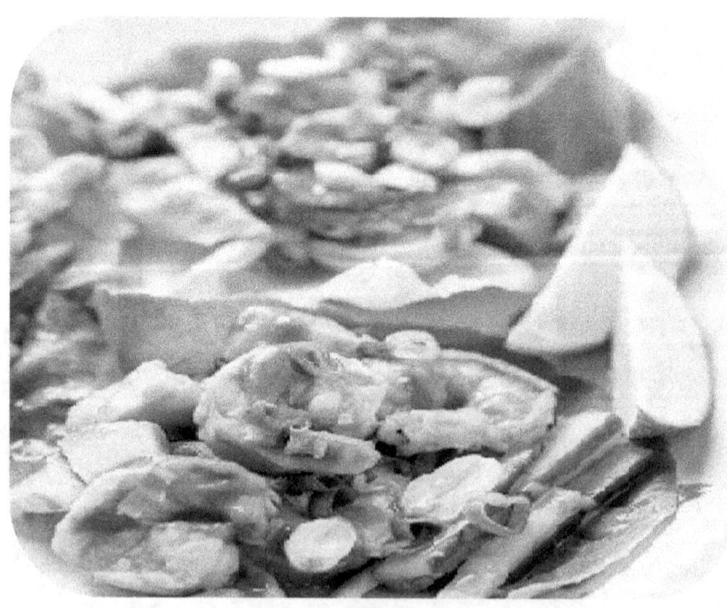

65

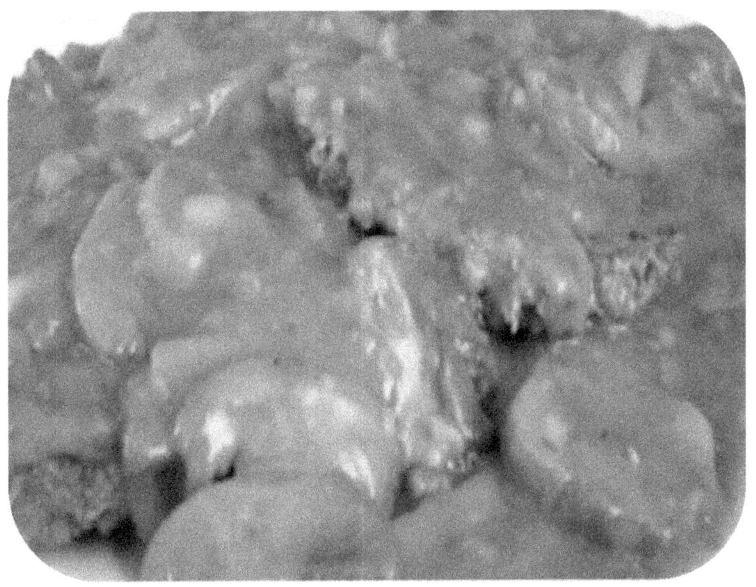

Thai Grilled Chicken

A Thai-inspired meal that includes marinated grilled chicken, coconut milk, curry, soy, minced garlic and more. So delicious!

Prep Time: 10minutes

Total Time: 10minutes

Servings: 4

Diet Phase: Solid food

Ingredients

1 1/2 lb. boneless, skinless chicken

Chopped parsley

1 cup coconut milk

2 teaspoon of curry paste

2 teaspoon of soy sauce

1 tablespoon of honey

1 teaspoon of minced garlic

Preparation:

1. Mix all the ingredients, (except for the chicken and parsley), in a zip lock bag.

2. Add chicken to the bag and shake to coat thoroughly. Place in the refrigerator overnight or for at least 4 hours to marinate.

3. Heat the grill.

4. Take out the chicken from the bag; pour the marinade into a saucepan. Use a paper towel to pat dry excess moisture on the chicken and spritz with non-stick cooking spray. Sprinkle with a little salt and place on the grill to

cook for 8 minutes on both sides on medium heat. Remove once internal temperature reads 160F. Do not overcook.

5. Now boil the marinade for 2 minutes.

6. Garnish chicken with parsley. Serve with rice. Pass the sauce.

7. *Make ahead*:

Place chicken in the refrigerator for up to 3 days. Enjoy the chicken hot, cold or at room temperature.

If enjoying hot, reheat in the microwave for a minute on high temperature. Reheat in the oven, if desired, at a temperature of 350F for 5 minutes.

*Nutrition Per Serving*Calories: 347kcal | Fat: 19g | Carbs: 9g | Protein: 34g| Fiber1 |Sodium: 327mg | Cholesterol 162mg

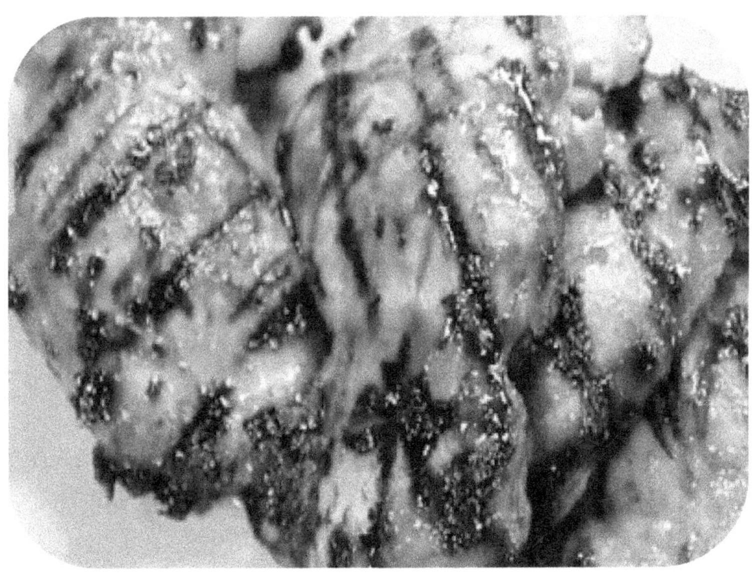

Balsamic Soy Salmon With Veggies

A healthy dinner option for the family!

Prep Time: 20minutes

Cook Time: 30minutes

Servings: 4

Diet Phase: Solid food

Ingredients:

For the salmon:

½ cup soy sauce

¼ cup olive oil

½ cup of balsamic vinegar

2 cloves garlic

2-12 oz. salmon fillets

Seasonings:

1 teaspoon garlic powder

1 teaspoon paprika

1 teaspoon onion powder

½ teaspoon pepper

1 teaspoon salt

2-12 oz. salmon fillets

Vegetables:

1 large carrot

5 oz. asparagus

5 oz. green beans

1 medium yellow squash

Olive oil, salt, pepper

<u>Preparation:</u>

1. Prepare your ingredients. Mince the garlic. Slice the carrots thinly. Trim the ends of the asparagus and then chop. Trim the ends of the green beans and chop. Chop the yellow squash.

2. Add together the soy sauce, olive oil, vinegar and garlic and mix to blend. Transfer to a square baking dish.

3. Coat 2 salmon fillets in the mixture and let it marinade for 2 hours in the refrigerator.

4. Preheat oven to 450°F.

5. Combine the onion powder, garlic powder, paprika, salt and pepper in a small bowl, and coat the remaining fillets evenly with the spices.

6. Place the salmon and the vegetables on a baking tray lined with parchment paper. Drizzle with oil and sprinkle with a little salt and pepper.

7. Bake 30 minutes.

8. ***Make ahead:*** Divide fish and veggies into 4 containers. Refrigerate for up to 3 days.

Nutrition Per Serving: *Calories: 608kcal | Fat: 42g | Carbs: 14g | Protein: 38g | Fiber 3g |*

Baked Tilapia

Spicy, tasty and healthy blackened Tilapia meal!

Prep Time: 5minutes

Cook Time: 10 minutes

Servings: 4

Diet Phase: Soft food

Ingredients

1 lb. (4) Tilapia fillets

2 tablespoons olive oil

Blackening Rub:

1 teaspoon salt

3 tablespoons paprika

1 teaspoon black pepper

1 tablespoons onion powder

1/4 teaspoon cayenne pepper

1 teaspoon oregano

1 teaspoon thyme

1/2 teaspoon garlic powder

Preparation:

1. Preheat oven to 425F.

2. Add together the salt, paprika, black pepper, onion powder, cayenne pepper, dry oregano, dry thyme, and garlic powder.

3. Line sheet pan with foil and brush it with oil, especially the area on the foil that the fish will be placed.

4. Rinse fish, pat dry and brush with oil. Rub the fillets with 1/3 of the mixed spices. Seal the rest in a container for future use.

5. Place on the greased pan and in the preheated oven. Cook for 10 minutes or thereabout or until internal temperature reads 145F.

Nutrition Per Serving *Calories: 178kcal | Fat: 10g | Carbs: 5g | Protein: 21g| Fiber1 | Sodium: 563mg | Cholesterol 40mg*

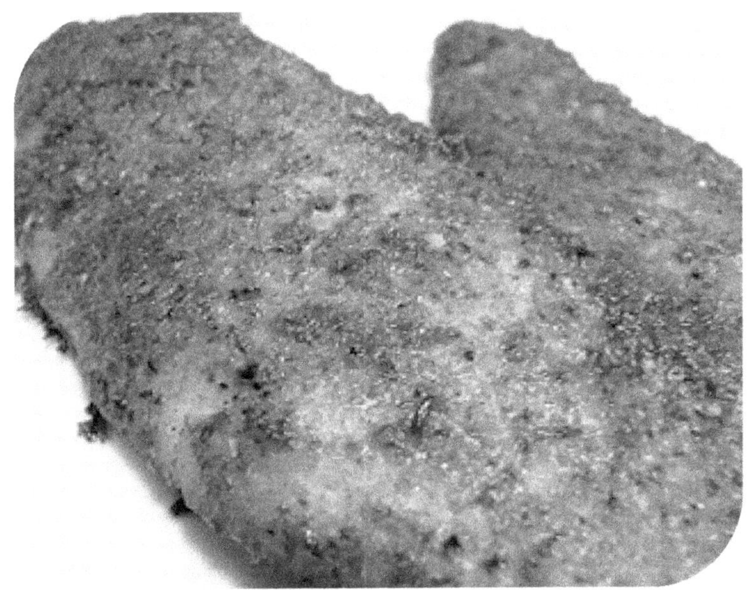

Slow Cooked Swiss Steak

Prep Time: 20minutes

Total Time: 4—4½ hours high

Servings: 6

Diet Phase: Soft food

<u>Ingredients</u>

1 large onion

1 green bell pepper

2 large carrots

1(2½ lb.) beef round steak

½ cup all-purpose flour

Salt and black pepper

2 tablespoons of canola oil, divided

1(14.5 oz.) can whole tomatoes, juice inclusive

1(14.5 oz.) can low-sodium beef broth

1 tablespoon of all-purpose flour

<u>Preparation:</u>

1. Slice the onions, slice the bell pepper, cut the carrots into 8 pieces, trim the round steak and cut into 6 pieces.

2. Place the onions, bell pepper and the carrots in a slow cooker.

3. Place each steak between 2 sheets of plastic wrap and pound.

4. Place the flour in a shallow disk, add salt and pepper and then dredge the steak in the flour; shake off excess.

5. Add a tablespoon of oil in a pan and heat over medium high. Brown steak in it for 6 minutes on both sides. Add more oil, when needed, to brown all steaks.

6. Place the browned steak on the layered vegetables in the slow cooker. Add the tomatoes and pour in the broth. Place the lid on and cook on high for 41/2 hours.

7. Remove steak to a plate, cover with foil. Remove vegetables to a plate. Remove 1/3 cup of liquid. Add the flour to the liquid to make a gravy.

8. Serve the swish steak with the vegetables and gravy.

Nutrition Per Serving *Calories: kcal | Fat: 14g | Carbs: 12g | Protein: 36g| Fiber2|Sodium: 267mg | Cholesterol 92mg*

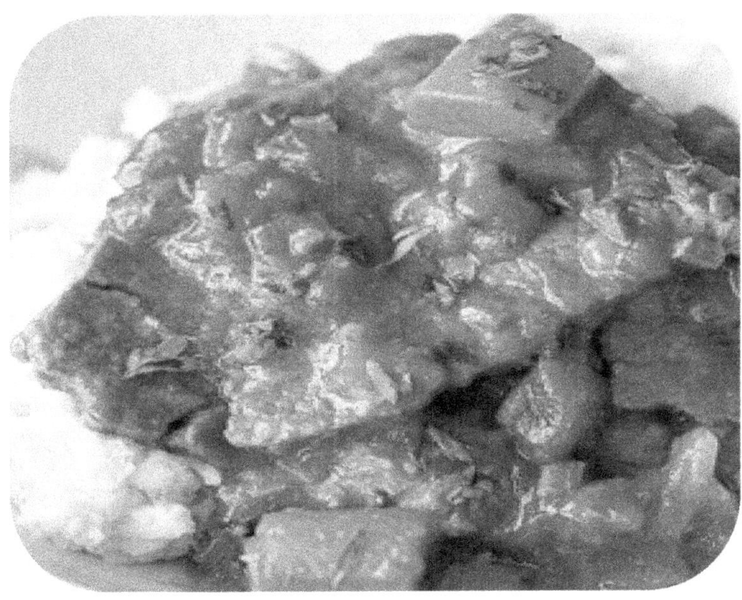

Creamy Fish Casserole

Prep Time: 10minutes

Cook Time: 30minutes

Servings:

Diet Phase: Soft food

Ingredients

2 tablespoons of canola oil

1 lb. broccoli, cut into florets

1 teaspoon of salt

¼ teaspoon of ground black pepper

6 scallions, chopped finely

2 tablespoons small capers

1 oz. butter

1½ lbs. salmon, in pieces

1¼ cups heavy whipping cream

1 tablespoons of Dijon mustard

1 tablespoons of dried parsley

3 oz. butter

Preparation:

1. Preheat your oven to 400°F.

2. Add the oil to a pan and fry the broccoli for 5 minutes until soft. Use medium high heat. Add the salt and pepper.

3. Add the scallions and capers. Cook 2 minutes and then transfer content to a greased baking dish.

4. Place the fish among the vegetables in the dish.

5. Combine the whipping cream, Dijon mustard and parsley in a small bowl and pour over the fish and vegetables. Place the butter slices on top.

6. Bake for 20 minutes. Remove fish if it flakes easily with a fork. Enjoy, if desired, with leafy greens.

Nutrition Per Serving *Calories: 797kcal | Fat: 67g |Net Carbs: 8g | Protein: 20g| Fiber5|Sodium: mg | Cholesterol mg*

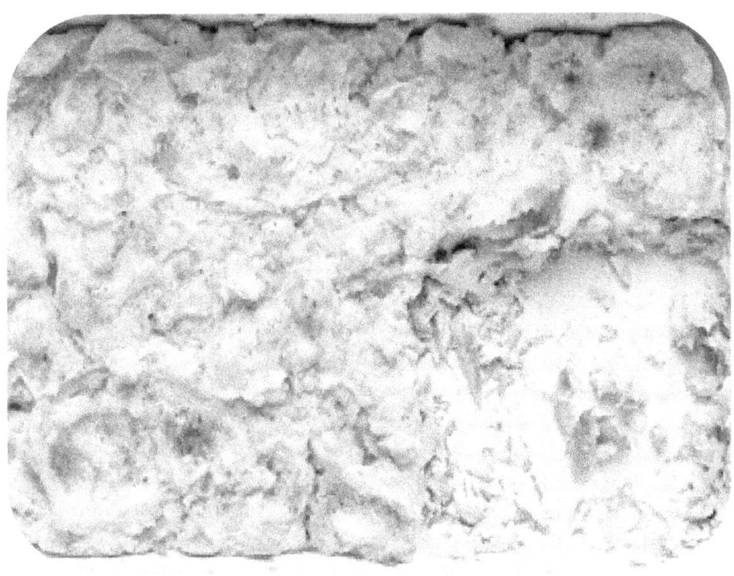

Quick Beef & Broccoli

Prep Time: 10 minutes

Cook Time: 10 minutes

Servings: 4

Diet Phase: Solid food

Ingredients:

1¼ cup of beef stock

2 tablespoons of horseradish sauce

50g unsalted cashews nuts

1 large head broccoli, cut into florets

14 oz. beef steak, cut into strips

4 sticks celery, sliced

1 tablespoons canola oil

2 tablespoons low-fat fromage frais

Pepper

Preparation:

1. In a skillet, heat the oil and add the nuts, tossing until lightly toasted and then setting aside.

2. Season the steak strips with pepper and stir-fry over a high heat until brown. Set aside. Tip the celery and broccoli into the pan and stir-fry 2 minutes.

3. Pour the stock, cover and simmer for another 2 minutes. Meanwhile, combine the fromage frais and horseradish well.

4. Return steak to pan and toss with the vegetable. Sprinkle over the nuts. Serve with the creamy horseradish.

Nutrition Per Serving *Calories: 269kcal | Fat: 14g | Net Carbs: 8g | Protein: 29g| Fiber3 | Carb 6g;*

Mushrooms Cajun Chicken

A great make-ahead dish!

Prep Time: 30minutes

Cook Time: 1 hr.15minutes

Servings: 5

Diet Phase: Stabilization

<u>Ingredients</u>

5chicken breasts pieces

1/4 cup extra virgin olive oil

1/2 cup flour

11/2 cups chopped celery

1-1/2 cups chopped onions

1 cup of chopped green bell peppers

1/2 cup red bell peppers

1 clove garlic, chopped

2-1/2 cups chicken broth

1/4 lb. baby carrots

4 oz. baby Bella mushrooms, sliced

1 bay leaf

2 teaspoons Worcestershire sauce

1/4 teaspoon cayenne pepper

2drops hot sauce

1/2 teaspoon seasoned salt

Parsley

Preparation:

1. Brown the chicken pieces in a large pan. Set aside.

2. Melt butter in a large heavy pan. Add flour, stir for a minute. Add onions, peppers, celery, and garlic. Cook and stir until softened.

3. Pour in the broth, stir and then add the carrots, mushrooms, cooked chicken and the rest of the seasoning. Do not add the parsley.

4. Cook for an hour. Remove the bay leaf. Serve, garnished with parsley.

5. *Make ahead*: Refrigerate for 24 hours. Favors meld and mix and dish generally tastes better.

Nutrition Per Serving *Calories: 522kcal | Fat: 18g | Carbs: 35g | Protein: 56g| Fiber7 | Sodium: 892 mg | Cholesterol 165mg*

Mushroom Pork Chops

Prep Time: 5 minutes

Cook Time: 40 minutes

Servings: 4

Ingredients:

1 onion, chopped

1/2 pound of fresh mushrooms, sliced

4 pork chops

Pinch of garlic salt

Salt & pepper to taste

1 can of condensed cream of mushroom soup (10.75-oz.)

Preparation:

1. Season pork chops with garlic salt, salt & pepper.

2. In a large skillet, brown pork chops over medium-high heat.

3. Add onions and mushrooms, sautéing for 1 minute then add the cream of mushroom soup.

4. Cover, reduce to medium-low heat then simmer 30 minutes to cook chops through.

Nutrition Per Serving *Calories: 210kcal | Fat: 9g |Carbs: 10g | Protein: 24g| Fiber1g|*

Slow Cooked Salsa Chicken

Prep Time: 1minute

Cook Time: 8 hours

Servings: 3 cups

Diet Phase: Soft food

<u>Ingredients</u>

2 (1 lbs. total) boneless, skinless chicken breasts

1 cup salsa of choice

Salt and pepper

<u>Preparation:</u>

1. Add chicken to a slow cooker, add the salsa and toss to coat chicken.

2. Cover and cook on high for 41/2 hours. If cooking low, cook for 8 hours.

3. Still in the slow cooker, shred the chicken and toss to thoroughly mix with the salsa and juices that's left. Serve and enjoy!

4. ***Make ahead***: store in an airtight container and place in the refrigerator for up to 5 days. Alternatively, freeze for 1-2 months.

Shrimp Scampi

Prep Time: 5 minutes

Cook Time: 10 minutes

Servings: 2

Diet Phase: Soft food

Ingredients

1 tablespoon of vegetable oil

1 lb. large shrimp, peeled &deveined

1/2 teaspoon of black pepper

1 teaspoon of sea salt

1/4 teaspoon of red pepper flakes, crushed

4 garlic cloves, minced

1/4 cup low-sodium chicken broth

Zest of 1/2 lemon

1/4 cup freshly squeezed lemon juice

1 lb. spiralized zucchini (from 2 large zucchinis)

1/4 cup Italian parsley, chopped

2 tablespoons of fresh parmesan, grated

Preparation:

1. Add the oil to a pan over medium- low heat.

2. Add the shrimp and then the salt, pepper and the red pepper flakes and cook for about 5 minutes until the shrimp is a little brown. Add the garlic and cook and stir for a minute.

3. Pour in the chicken broth, zest of lemon, lemon juice and the zucchini noodles (spiralized zucchini).

4. Boil and cook for a minute. Sprinkle with the parsley and the parmesan and serve.

5. *Make ahead*:

Spiralize zucchini and store refrigerated in an airtight container for up to 5 days. Freeze the shrimp and stock in a container.

When ready to cook, reheat shrimp in a microwave for a few minutes. Alternatively, reheat in skillet, together with the zucchini noodles until heated through.

Nutrition Per Serving*Calories: 354kcal | Fat: 11g | Carbs: 12g | Protein: 36g | Fiber6 | Sodium: 2746mg | Cholesterol 571mg*

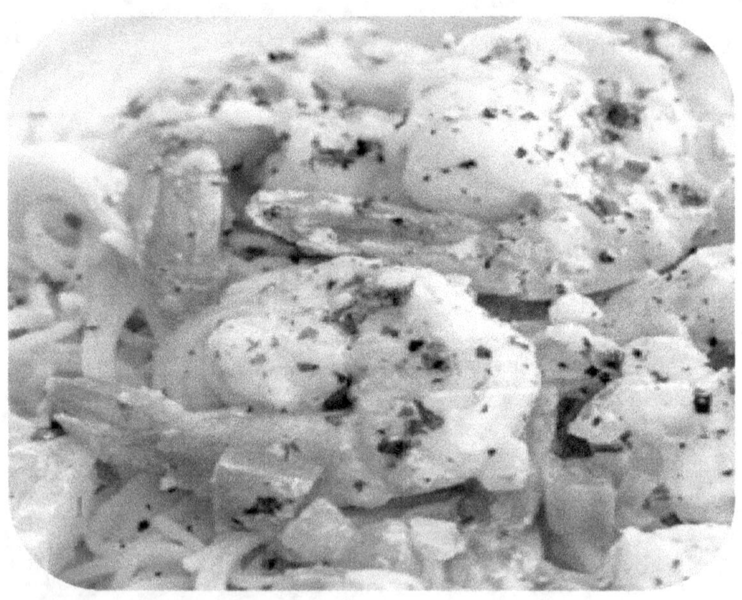

Easy Chicken & Spinach Meatballs

Prep Time: 10minutes

Cook Time: 30 minutes

Servings: 6; 18 meatballs

Diet Phase: Soft food

Ingredients

1 lb. ground chicken

10-oz box frozen spinach

2 tablespoons fresh basil

2 large garlic cloves, minced

1/2 medium onion

2 eggs, beaten

1/4 cup breadcrumbs

1/4 cup of shredded Parmesan cheese

1/4 teaspoon black pepper

1/2 teaspoon of salt

Preparation:

1. Thaw frozen spinach completely, wrap in dish towel and wring out excess moisture. Once drained, chop. Chop the fresh basil and the onion. Mince the garlic.

2. Preheat oven to 350°F.

3. Combine all the ingredients in a bowl, form into balls and place on a greased baking sheet. Bake for 30 minutes at 350°F

4. ***Make ahead***: store in an airtight container and refrigerate for up to 3 days. To freeze: cool and store in an airtight container. Freeze for up to 4 months.

Nutrition Per Serving (3meatballs)*Calories: 206kcal | Fat: 10.6g |Carbs: 7.3g | Protein: 21.1g| Fiber1.9|Sodium: 461mg | Cholesterol 132.7mg*

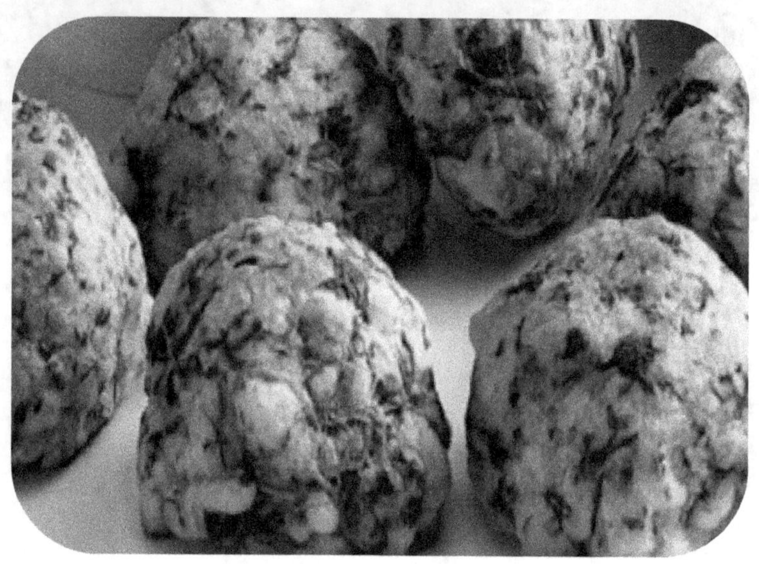

Sautéed Spinach And Leeks

Simple ingredients loaded with delicious flavor, enjoy with a simple dinner or eat with browned meat!

Prep Time: 5 minutes

Cook Time: 8minutes

Servings: 4

Diet Phase: Soft food

Ingredients

1 teaspoon olive oil

1 medium leek

2 garlic cloves, minced

1 8 oz. bag spinach

Salt and pepper

Preparation:

1. Clean the leek, trim, slice and then toss in water to remove dirt or sand. Gently lift from the dirty water onto a colander and let it sit for 2 minutes.

2. Sauté the leeks for 3 minutes or until soft. Add the garlic and cook for 30 seconds. Add the spinach and cook for 3 minutes or thereabouts.

3. Season with salt and pepper.

Nutrition Per Serving *Calories: 42kcal | Fat: 2g |Carbs: 5g | Protein: 36g| Fiber2|Sodium: 1mg | Cholesterol 1mg*

Limy Spicy Garlicky Chicken

Prep Time: 10minutes

Cook Time: 17 minutes

Servings: 4

Ingredients:

4 chicken breast halves, boneless& skinless

1/4 teaspoon cayenne pepper

1/8 teaspoon of paprika

1/8 teaspoon of onion powder

1/4 teaspoon of garlic powder

1/4 teaspoon of dried parsley

1/4 teaspoon of dried thyme

3/4 teaspoon of salt

1/4 teaspoon of black pepper

2 tablespoons butter

1 tablespoon olive oil

2 teaspoons garlic powder

3 tablespoons of lime juice

Preparation:

1. In a small bowl, add together1/4 teaspoon garlic, paprika, onion powder, cayenne pepper, powder, thyme, salt, parsley and black pepper.

2. Season chicken generously on both sides with spices mixture.

3. Melt butter and olive oil in a skillet over medium heat. Cook the chicken about 6 minutes per side in hot oil until golden brown.

4. Add 2 teaspoons of garlic powder and lime juice. Cook, stirring frequently for another 5 minutes.

Nutrition Per Serving *Calories: 220kcal | Fat: 11g |Carbs: 3g | Protein: 30g| Fiber1g|*

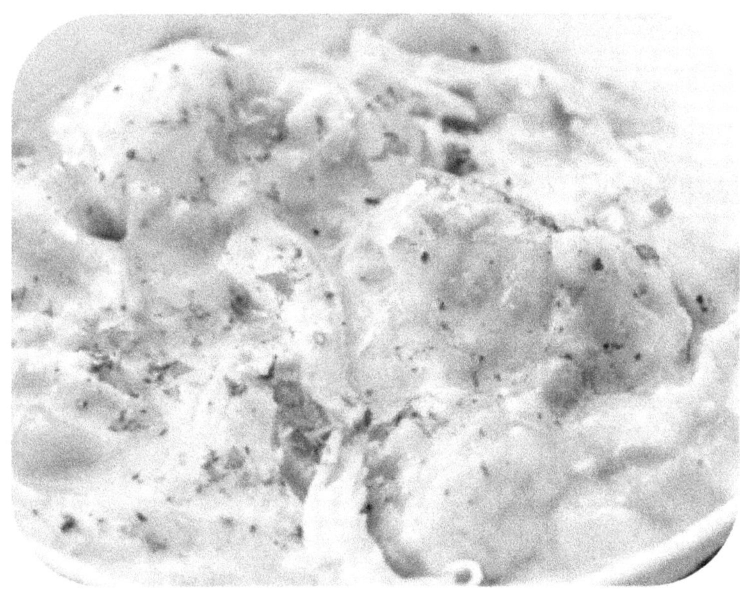

Chicken and dumplings

Chicken And Dumplings

Warm and hearty chicken and vegetables dinner for the whole family.

Prep Time: 20 minutes

Cook Time: 1 hr. 40 minutes

Servings: 4

Diet Phase: Soft food

<u>Ingredients</u>

<u>Stew:</u>

1 lb. (4)chicken thighs

Freshly ground black pepper

Salt

1 teaspoon of canola oil

1large onion

1largecarrot

1 celery rib

1 tablespoon of apple cider vinegar

3 cups of low salt chicken broth

1/4 teaspoon dried thyme leaves

8 oz. chicken wings

1/8 cup minced parsley leaves

<u>Dumplings:</u>

½ cup all-purpose flour

½ cup whole wheat flour

½ teaspoon sugar

½ teaspoon salt

1/4teaspoon baking soda

½ cup of cold buttermilk

2 tablespoons melted unsalted butter

1 small egg white

Preparation:

1. Season the chicken thigh with salt and pepper. Cook the chicken in heated oil for about 10 minutes on both sides. Remove to a plate. Leave just a teaspoon of fat in the pot.

2. Cook the onions, the carrot and celery in the pot for 7 minutes or thereabout until softened. Add the apple cider vinegar gently. Pour in the broth and add the thyme. Return chicken and juices to pot. Add the chicken wings. Cover and bring to simmer for 55 minutes.

3. Turn off heat. Remove chicken thighs and wings with tongs and cool slightly on a plate. Use a spoon to skim fat from the stew. Remove meat from bones and shred. Add boneless and skinless meat back to the pot.

4. In a large bowl, combine the flours, the sugar, baking soda and salt. In a medium bowl, add together the butter and buttermilk and then add the egg white, whisking in. Add the buttermilk mixture to the flour mixture, stirring well.

5. Simmer stew again, add the parsley. Add batter in gentle scoops to the top of the stew. Cover and simmer until dumplings are twice its size. Serve!

6. ***Make ahead***: after removing the chicken from pot, cool and remove the bones. Place tightly in a container and refrigerate for up to 2 days. Refrigerate broth in the pot or Dutch oven. When ready to cook, skim the fat from the broth, return the chicken to the stew. Continue with the recipe to simmer it. Prepare the dumplings.

Nutrition Per Serving *Calories: 519kcal | Fat: 28g |Carbs:29g | Protein: 35g| Fiber3|Sodium: 1221mg | Cholesterol 126mg*

Chicken Enchilada Casserole

Easy, creamy, layered chicken enchilada casserole packed with flavor and texture.

Prep Time: 25 minutes

Cook Time: 40 minutes

Servings: 4

Diet Phase: Stabilization

Ingredients

3 cups Rotisserie chicken, shredded

1 (15 oz.) can pinto beans rinsed & drained

3 cups of shredded cheese

15 corn tortillas, halved

Sauce

2 tablespoons of unsalted butter

2 tablespoon extra-virgin olive oil

1/2 cup chopped onion

4 cloves garlic, minced

1/4 cup of all-purpose flour

2 cups low sodium chicken broth

1 cup salsa verde

1 4 oz. can mild diced green chili, un-drained

1 teaspoon of chicken bouillon

1 teaspoon of ground cumin

1 teaspoon of salt

1/2 teaspoon cayenne pepper

1 cup of sour cream

Preparation:

1. Preheat oven to 350F. Spritz baking dish lightly with cooking spray.

2. Add butter to a saucepan, add olive oil and melt it over medium heat. Sauté onion for 3 minutes and add the flour and garlic. Cook for 2 minutes.

3. Lower heat and add the broth, salsa Verde, the green chilies, bullion and the spices, mix well, let it boil, then simmer to thicken. Remove; add the sour cream and mix to combine.

4. Remove ½ cup of the enchilada sauce and spread it in the bottom of the greased baking dish evenly.

5. Add the chicken and beans to the sauce in the pan.

6. Place 10 tortilla halves onto the sauce; fill the center with the other halves. Add 1/3 of the chicken mixture evenly,1 cup of cheese. Do same with another tortilla layer: 1/3 chicken mixture, and then 1 cup cheese. And then the final layer.

7. Cover with foil and bake for 20 minutes at 350F. Take out the foil and bake 20 more minutes. Remove pan and add toppings as desired.

8.***Make ahead*:** Cover enchilada with foil tightly and refrigerate for up to 24 hours. When ready to cook, increase baking time by 10 minutes.

To freeze casserole: it is advisable to char the tortillas to prevent it from getting soft on time. Cool and wrap tightly with plastic wrap, and then with foil.

When ready to eat, thaw in the fridge for 24 hours. Bake covered 30 minutes at 350F degrees. Remove foil and bake 20 more minutes.

Nutrition Per Serving *Calories: 1043kcal | Fat: 51g |Carbs: 124g | Protein: 60g| Fiber7g|Sodium: 2088mg | Cholesterol 108mg*

Chicken Parmesan

Prep Time: 15 minutes

Cook Time: 40minutes

Servings: 4

Diet Phase:Soft food

Ingredients

1 lb. raw chicken breast

1 large egg

2/3cup panko bread crumbs

2 tablespoons of grated parmesan cheese

¾ teaspoon of Italian seasoning

½ teaspoon garlic powder

1 (8 oz.) can tomato sauce

¾ cup mozzarella cheese

Preparation:

1. Preheat your oven to 375F.

2. Pound the chicken to 1/2-inch thickness, or thereabouts.

3. Whisk egg in a bowl.

4. Add together in a separate bowl; the parmesan, the Italian seasoning and the garlic powder.

5. Dip each breast in egg, and coat in the bread crumb mixture. Place on a greased baking sheet and bake for 20 minutes, flipping halfway through. Let it cool for 30 minutes.

6. ***Make ahead***: Freeze in re-sealable bags that have smaller bags of the tomato sauce and the mozzarella cheese. When ready to eat, thaw overnight in the refrigerator and reheat for 20 minutes at 375F. Top the chicken with the tomato sauce, and mozzarella. Bake to melt cheese for 3 minutes.

Nutrition Per Serving *Calories: 258.9kcal | Fat: 8.7g | Carbs: 10.7g | Protein: 33g| Fiber 1.3g| Sodium 602mg| Cholesterol 126mg*

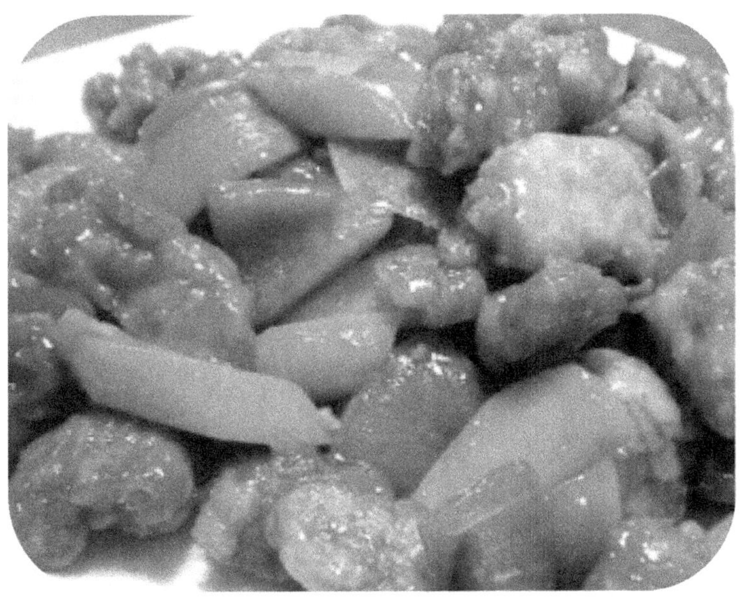

Sweet and sour pork

Sweet And Sour Pork

Authentic sweet and sour pork meal with a sweet tangy sauce.

Prep Time: 10 minutes

Cook Time: 10 minutes

Servings: 2

Diet Phase: Stabilization

Ingredients

1/2 lb. pork tenderloin

1/2 red bell pepper

1/2 green bell pepper

2 stalks scallions

1 piece pineapple ring

1 clove garlic

Vegetable oil

For the marinade:

1/2 teaspoon cornstarch

1 teaspoon soy sauce

1/2 teaspoon rice wine

For the Batter:

4 tablespoons of all-purpose flour

2 tablespoon cornstarch

1/2 teaspoon baking soda

1/2 egg

1/2 cup of water

1 teaspoon olive oil

1 pinch salt

For the sauce (sweet and sour):

1 1/2 tablespoons tomato ketchup

1 teaspoon of plum sauce

1/8 teaspoon Chinese rice vinegar

1/2 teaspoon Worcestershire Sauce

1 teaspoon cornstarch

1 teaspoon oyster sauce

1 teaspoon sugar

2 tablespoons water

Preparation:

1. Prepare ingredients: cut the pork tenderloin into bite size pieces; cut the peppers into pieces; cut the white part of the scallions into 2 inch length; cut the pineapple into small pieces; finely chop the garlic.

2. Add the pork tenderloins and marinade ingredients together in a bowl and let it rest for 20 minutes.

3. Combine the sauce ingredients together and set to one side.

4. Combine the flour, cornstarch and baking soda in a bowl, strain and add to the egg, the water and cooking oil in another bowl, whisking to thicken into a batter.

5. Place the marinated pork pieces to the batter and coat thoroughly.

6. Add the cooking oil to a deep pan and fry the pork pieces until golden brown; drain on paper towels.

7. Add the garlic to heated oil in a wok and cook for a few minutes. Add the bell peppers and the chopped pineapples. Cook and stir 1-2 minutes and then add the sauce.

8. Once sauce thicken, add the pork to the wok and stir. Add the chopped scallions, stir for a while and then turn off heat.

9. Serve with rice.

Nutrition Per Serving*Calories: 402kcal | Fat: 8g |Carbs: 52g | Protein: 29g| Fiber3|Sodium: 758mg | Cholesterol 115mg*

Slow Cooker Chicken Chili Verde

Prep Time: 5 minutes

Cook Time: 4 hrs.

Servings: 4

Diet Phase: Soft food

Ingredients

1 lb. boneless skinless chicken thighs

2 tablespoons cornstarch

15 oz. jar salsa verde

2 cups of chicken broth

Preparation:

1. Place the chicken in the slow cooker. Sprinkle chicken with cornstarch. Pour in the broth and salsa.

2. Place the lid on and cook for 4 hours on high or for 8 hours on low. Remove, shred and place back in the slow cooker.

3. Serve as desired over rice or vegetable noodles.

4.*Make ahead*: store, ingredients in a Ziploc bag and refrigerate for up to 3 days or freeze in a freezer safe container for up to 3 months. To cook, thaw first. For leftovers, cool and store, refrigerated for up to 3 days.

*Nutrition Per Serving*Calories: 217kcal | Fat: 7g | Carbs: 12g | Protein: 24g| Fiber2 | Sodium: 901mg | Cholesterol 108mg

Slow Cooker Sweet and Sour Pork

A slow cooked version of your favorite dish of pork, bell peppers and pineapple rings to prepare for the whole family; ahead of time!

Prep Time: 15 minutes

Cook Time: 8 hours 15 minutes

Servings: 8

Diet Phase: Stabilization

Ingredients

1/2 cup sugar

1/2 cup brown sugar

1/2 cup of chicken broth

3 tablespoons lemon juice

1/3 cup white vinegar

3 tablespoons low sodium soy sauce

3 tablespoons tomato paste

1/4 teaspoon ground ginger

1/2 teaspoon garlic powder

1/4 teaspoon ground black pepper

1 1/2 pounds boneless pork loin chops, cubed

1 large green pepper, cut into pieces

1 large onion, cut into pieces

8 ounces pineapple chunks, drained

3 tablespoons cornstarch

1/3 cup of chicken broth

<u>Preparation:</u>

1. Add all the ingredients together in a slow cooker; but add the pork, green pepper, onion and pineapple last. Stir well.

2. Cover and cook for 6 to 8 hours on low.

3. Add together the cornstarch and broth to smoothness and add to the cooking juices, stirring well.

4. Cover and cook for 15 minutes to thicken sauce.

Nutrition Per Serving *Calories: 272kcal | Fat: 3g | Carbs: 41g | Protein: 20g | Fiber1 | Sodium: 385mg | Cholesterol 56mg*

Taco Salad Bowls

A great make-ahead recipe with seasoned beef, lettuce, cheese, and more!

Prep Time: 10minutes

Cook Time: 10 minutes

Servings: 4

Diet Phase: Stabilization

Ingredients

1 lb. ground beef

1 teaspoon cumin

1 teaspoon chili Powder

1/2 teaspoon garlic powder

1/2 teaspoon onion salt

Salt and pepper

6cups romaine lettuce, chopped

1/3 cup of ranch dressing

1 tablespoon adobo sauce

1/2 onion, diced

1/2 cup of diced tomatoes

1/2 jalapeno, deseed and diced finely

1 tablespoon cilantro, finely chopped

1/2 cup of shredded Mexican blend cheese

Preparation:

1. Combine onions, cilantro, tomatoes, and the jalapenos in a bowl. Set aside. Add the ranch dressing and the adobo sauce together and set aside.

2. Add the ground beef to a pan and add the cumin, chili powder, garlic powder, onion powder and season with salt and pepper. Sauté until brown.

3. Assemble fresh salad, add lettuce to bottom of bowl, top with ground beef, shredded cheese, tomato and onion mixture (pico), and toppings as desired such as sliced avocado, sour cream or crushed tortilla chips. Drizzle with the chipotle ranch dressing

4. ***Make ahead***:

Divide lettuce between 4Ziploc bags. Divide the cheese between 4 jello shot cups. Divide the sauce between 4 jello shot cups. Divide the pico between 4 jello shot cups.

Place condiments and the lettuce in 4 meal prep containers, leave space for the ground beef. Fill space with ground beef. Cover and refrigerate.

When ready to eat, remove the condiments cups and lettuce from container, microwave the ground beef. Add lettuce and condiments to the container including any additional toppings and serve.

Nutrition Per Serving *Calories: 409kcal | Fat: 29g | Carbs: 12g | Protein: 31g | Fiber1g | Sodium: 661mg | Cholesterol 89mg*

Chicken, Sweet Potatoes, Kale And Cranberries

Prep Time: 15 minutes

Cook Time: 15minutes

Servings: 4

Diet Phase: Solid food

Ingredients

1 tablespoon extra-virgin olive oil

2 medium sweet potatoes

3/4 teaspoon salt

1/4 teaspoon ground black pepper

1 large bunch kale

1 tablespoon of minced garlic

2 chicken breasts, cooked &diced or shredded (about 3 cups)

1 1/2 tablespoons balsamic vinegar

1 tablespoon chopped fresh thyme

1 tablespoon chopped fresh sage

1/4 cup dried cranberries

4 oz. goat cheese

Preparation:

1, Scrub potatoes, peel, and cut into 1/2-inches. Stem kale and chop roughly to get about 8 cups.

2. Add oil to a large and deep pan and heat over medium high. Add the sweet potatoes to the hot oil, sprinkle with salt and pepper and cook and stir for 3 minutes to soften.

3. Add the kale, gradually, and cook and stir until wilted in the large pan. Cook and stir another 5 minutes to soften and then add the garlic. Cook and stir for a minute.

4. Now add the chicken, stir and then add the vinegar, sage, the thyme, and the cranberries.

5. Crumble½ cheese over the top, stir to melt and make creamy. Taste for seasonings and adjust as desired. Sprinkle the remaining cheese over the top.

6. Enjoy with brown rice, quinoa or cauliflower rice.

Nutrition Per Serving *Calories: 509kcal | Fat: 16g |Carbs: 35g | Protein: 59g| Fiber9g| | Cholesterol 148mg*

Quinoa With Eggplant& Chickpea

Prep Time: 15minutes

Cook Time: 55minutes

Servings: 3

Diet Phase: Solid food

Ingredients

Quinoa Mix:

½ cup of rinsed quinoa

1cup of water

18- ounce can of chickpeas, drained, rinsed, chopped

1/4 teaspoon cumin

1/4 teaspoon of cinnamon

1/4teaspoon allspice

1/8 teaspoon black pepper

1/8teaspoon salt

Eggplant Mix:

1 tablespoons canola oil

1 garlic clove, minced

1 small onion, chopped

1 large eggplant, washed &chopped coarsely

1/8 teaspoon black pepper

1/8teaspoon salt

1/3 cup of pine nuts

½ tablespoon of lemon juice

Preparation:

1. Boil water. Set heat to low, add the quinoa, stir, cover pot and simmer 15 minutes to enable quinoa absorb all the water. Fluff.

2. Add the chickpeas to the pot of quinoa. Add the cinnamon, allspice, cumin, and salt and pepper, and stir to blend.

3. Sauté onion in hot oil for 5 minutes until translucent. Stir in garlic; stir. Add the eggplant, ½ of the salt and pepper, uncover and cook until eggplant is soft. That should be between 7 to 8 minutes. Add the pine nuts, stir, add the lemon juice and stir again. Set to one side.

4. Spread ½ of quinoa mix to greased baking dish and spread the eggplant mixture it. Add the remaining quinoa mixture on top and bake for 30 minutes350F degrees until heated through.

Nutrition Per Serving *Calories: 462kcal | Fat: 22g | Carbs: 53g | Protein: 18g | Fiber16g |* Sodium 601mg *| Cholesterol 0mg*

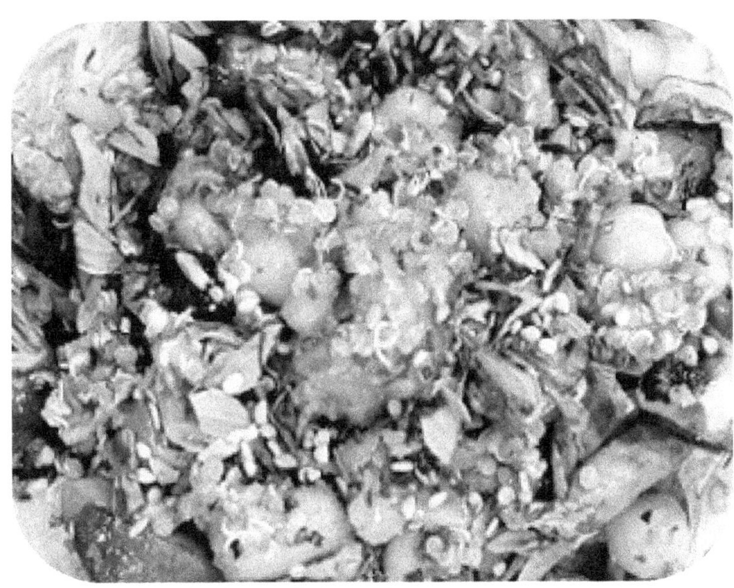

Make Ahead Taco Casserole

Prep Time: 10minutes

Cook Time: 45minutes

Servings: 6

Diet Phase: Soft food

<u>Ingredients</u>

1 lb. lean ground beef

1 small yellow onion, diced

2 tablespoons of taco seasoning

1 lb. refried beans

¾ cup of sour cream

2 cups of shredded cheese (cheddar &Monterey Jack)

1/3 cup tomatoes, diced

¼ cup black olives, sliced

¾ cup tortilla chips

1/3 cup shredded lettuce

<u>Preparation:</u>

1. Preheat your oven to 350F.

2. Cook the ground beef and onions in a large pan until thoroughly cooked. Drain excess and then pour in ¾ cup of water and add the taco seasoning. Let it boil.

3. Lower heat and let it simmer with occasional stirring for 5 minutes; turn off heat.

4. Spread the refried beans in a casserole dish evenly layered. Add the sour cream on the refried beans, spreading over it. Top with the mixture of cooked ground beef and then the cheese.

5.***Make ahead***: cool, cover the dish and refrigerate. When ready to cook, bake, with the lid on, for 25 minutes. Uncover and bake for 5 more minutes.

6. Add toppings (tomatoes, black olives or crunchy toppings like tortilla chips and more cheese, if desired). Bake for 8 minutes without covering.

7. Garnish with shredded lettuce and green onions, if desired. Serve!

Nutrition Per Serving *Calories: 547kcal | Fat: 38g | Carbs: 24g | Protein: 28g| Fiber5g| Sodium: 1273mg| Cholesterol 108mg|*

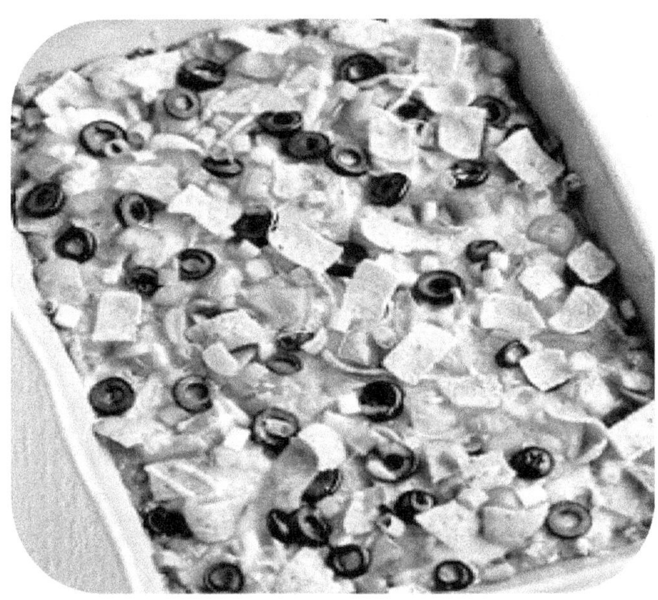

Turkey Rice Bowl

Prep Time: 10minutes

Cook Time: 30minutes

Servings: 5

Diet Phase: Soft food

Ingredients

3 tablespoons olive oil

1 (20-oz.) pkg. Italian Turkey Sausage Links

1 teaspoon of minced garlic

1 pepper

2 bell peppers

1 medium yellow onion

1 teaspoon of salt

1/4 teaspoon of cumin power

Cauliflower Rice:

1/3 cup of warm water

1/3 cup of cilantro, minced

1 teaspoon of kosher salt

1 small cauliflower

3 tablespoons of lime juice

Preparation:

1. Prepare ingredients: cut the turkey sausage links into coins; slice the peppers thinly; slice the yellow onion thinly; mince the cilantro; cut the cauliflower into small florets.

2. Heat 2 tablespoons of oil in a large skillet set over medium heat, add sausage coins and cook for about 5 minutes per side until cooked through and browned. Remove from heat and set aside in a bowl.

3. Add the remaining tablespoon of olive oil to the skillet and heat. Add garlic and sauté for a few minutes until fragrant.

4. Next, add bell pepper, poblano pepper, cumin, onions and salt. Cook for a few minutes stirring occasionally until soft.

5. Add sausage to the pan and mix with the veggies, reduce heat to low and simmer for a few minutes.

6. Meanwhile, add florets to a blender and pulse until it resembles rice sticks.

7. Transfer to a microwavable bowl, add water, salt and stir. Place in the microwave and heat on high for 5 minutes.

8. Remove from heat; add cilantro, lime juice and mix. Serve with the turkey sausage.

Nutrition Per Serving *Calories: 321 kcal | Fat: 19g | Carbs: 15g | Protein: 23g | Fiber 5g | Sodium: 767mg | Cholesterol 70mg |*

Chicken With Rosemary And Mushrooms

A quick enjoyable no make-ahead family dinner!

Prep Time: 5minutes

Cook Time: 20minutes

Servings: 4-6

Diet Phase: Solid food

Ingredients

3 tablespoons unsalted butter

16 oz. white button mushrooms

3 garlic cloves, minced

1 teaspoon fresh rosemary or 1 1/2 teaspoons dried

1/4 teaspoon salt

1/2 cup low-sodium chicken stock

2 teaspoon all-purpose flour

1/1/2 lb. boneless, skinless chicken

Preparation:

1. Melt butter in deep skillet and then add the sliced mushrooms, the minced garlic, rosemary and the kosher salt.

2. Cook to brown mushrooms for 5 minutes. Add the chicken stock and the flour and cook and whisk to slightly thicken for 2 minutes. Remove all to a bowl.

3. Place chicken in the skillet and cook over medium heat. If not enough oil in pat, add more butter. Cook for about 15 minutes on both sides. Chicken is done when an internal temperature reads 165°F.

4. Add back the mushroom and sauce to the pan and cook for a minute. Enjoy warm.

Nutrition Per Serving *Calories: 216kcal | Fat: 9.2g | Carbs: 4.4g | Protein: 28.6g| Fiber0.8g| Sodium: 181.4mg| Cholesterol 98.6mg*

Make Ahead Cajun Chicken Alfredo Pasta

Prep Time: 5minutes

Cook Time: 15minutes

Servings: 4

Diet Phase: Solid food

Ingredients

8 oz. pasta

2 tablespoons butter

3 garlic cloves, minced

1 lb. boneless skinless chicken breasts, cut into pieces

2 teaspoons of Cajun seasoning

4 oz. low fat cream cheese, softened, cut into pieces

1 cup skim milk

3/4 cup fresh parmesan cheese, grated

1/2 teaspoon ground black pepper

1/2 teaspoon salt

Preparation:

1. Melt butter and add the garlic. Cook and then add the chicken. Add the Cajun seasoning and cook for a few minutes until the chicken is almost cooked.

2. Stir in the milk and the cream cheese, and cook for 2 minutes.

3. Cool and refrigerate for up to 2 days.

4. When ready to eat, cook pasta until al dente. Drain, rinse and set aside. Reheat the chicken sauce and then add the pasta and the cheese to it. Season with salt and pepper. Serve!

Nutrition Per Serving *Calories: 661kcal | Fat: 27g | Carbs: 58g | Protein: 46g| Fiber5g| Sodium: 930mg| Cholesterol 141mg|*

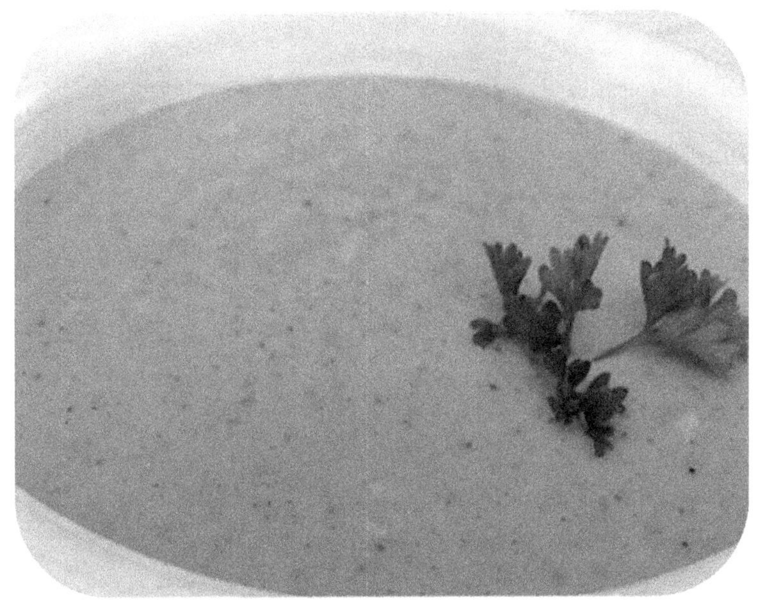

Simple Chicken Broth

Prep Time: 10 minutes

Cook Time: 45 minutes

Servings: 8 cups

Diet Phase: Clear Liquid

<u>Ingredients</u>

1 chicken breast

1/2 teaspoon salt

1 teaspoon extra virgin olive oil

1 large red onion, peeled, chopped

2 stalks celery, trimmed chopped

2 medium carrots, peeled, chopped

1/4 cup parsley, chopped

1 teaspoon of whole black peppercorns

2 bay leaves

12 cups of water

<u>Preparation:</u>

1. Sprinkle the chicken with sea salt.

2. Cook the chicken in a large stockpot for 4 minutes. Cook with the skin side down until browned.

3. Add the carrots, onions, and celery in the pot and cook another 4 minutes, with occasional stirring.

4. Add the peppercorns, parsley and the bay leaf. Pour the water and bring to a boil gently. Let the heat be high. Reduce heat and simmer for 25 minutes. Use a spoon to skim fat off the top of the broth.

4. Remove the chicken, discard the skin and set aside meat for future use.

5. *Make ahead*: Let the broth cool completely and then store refrigerated in an air-tight bowl. Store for up to a week or in the freezer for up to 6 months.

6. Before using, discard the bay leaf and peppercorns. Serving Size: 1 cup.

Nutrition Per Serving *Calories: 40kcal | Fat: 2g | Carbs: 4g | Protein: 0g| Fiber1g| Sodium: 125mg| Cholesterol 1mg|*

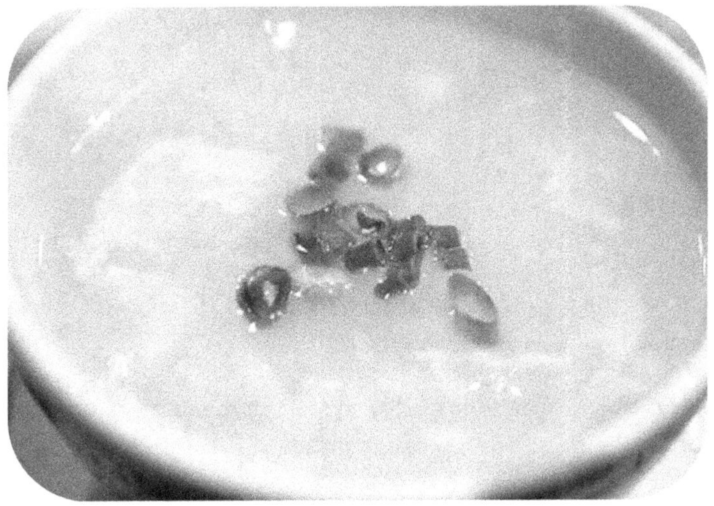

Egg drop soup

Egg Drop Soup

Prep Time: 5 minutes

Cook Time: 5minutes

Servings: 1

Diet Phase: Clear Liquid

Ingredients:

1 cup of chicken broth

1 tablespoon bacon fat

½ cube chicken bouillon

2 eggs

1 teaspoon chili garlic paste

Preparation:

1. Combine the chicken broth, bacon fat and bouillon cube in a pan and bring to boil on medium- high heat.

2. Add the chicken paste and stir thoroughly. Remove from heat.

3. Whisk the egg into the steaming broth and stir to mix. Let it sit for a couple of minutes and then serve!

4. ***Make ahead:*** pack properly and store in the refrigerator for up to 5days. Store in the freezer for up to a month.

Nutrition Per Serving: *Calories: 289kcal | Fat: 23.24g |Net Carbs: 2.92g | Protein: 15.3g*

Broccoli & Cheese Soup

Easy, healthy and super cheesy!

Prep Time: 2 minutes

Cook Time: 20minutes

Servings: 4

Diet Phase: Full Liquid

Ingredients:

2 cups broccoli, cut into florets

2 cloves garlic, minced

13/4 cups of vegetable broth

½ cup heavy cream

11/2 cups cheddar cheese

Preparation:

1. Sauté the garlic in a large pot until fragrant.

2. Add the vegetable broth, broccoli and heavy cream. Raise the heat and bring to a boil. Lower heat and let it simmer until broccoli is tender. This should take between 10 to 20 minutes.

3. Gradually add the cheddar cheese ½ cup at a time; stir continuously and keep stirring on very low simmer until melted. Repeat process of adding another ½ cup until all the cheese is used up.

4. Once cheese melts, remove immediately.

Nutrition Per Serving: *Calories: 291 kcal | Fat: 25g | Net Carbs: 4g | Protein: 13g*

Italian Shrimp And Veggie Soup

A large batch of low-calorie hearty soup to make-ahead for the family.

Prep Time: 15 minutes

Cook Time: 35minutes

Servings: 7

Diet Phase: Soft food

Ingredients

1 bulb fennel

1 medium onions

2 stalk celery

3 garlic clove

3 tablespoons of olive oil

1 teaspoon of dried marjoram

1/2 teaspoon of red pepper flakes

1/4 teaspoon of salt

1 zucchini

1 spinach

5 cup water

14.5 oz. can diced tomatoes, no salt added

1 Shrimp

15 oz. can great northern beans

Preparation:

1. Chop the fennel, onion, celery and clove. Cut the zucchini to pieces and add to a pot. Add the marjoram, the pepper flakes and the salt and cook for 15 minutes, stirring occasionally.

2. Once vegetables soften, add the zucchini and spinach and cook and stir for 10 minutes. Now add the tomatoes and the water and let it simmer, covered for about 10 minutes, until the veggies are tender.

3. Add the shrimp, stir and then add beans and simmer, gently with the lid off for about 2 minutes.

4. ***Make ahead:*** Freeze for up to a month. Reheat shrimp gently until tender.

Nutrition Per Serving: *Calories: 260kcal | Fat: 6.7g |Net Carbs: 31.8g | Protein: 20.4g |Dietary Fiber: 9.5 g| Cholesterol: 94.3 mg| Sodium: 516.5 mg*

Chicken Corn Chowder

Prep Time: 10 minutes

Cook Time: 40 minutes

Servings: 3

Diet Phase: Soft food

Ingredients:

3 bacon strips, cut into small pieces

1 large chicken breast, cut into small pieces

1 stick celery, chopped

1/4 medium onion, chopped

1/1 -2 tablespoons of flour

1 garlic clove, minced

2 cups chicken stock

1 cup of frozen corn

½ cup heavy/whipping cream

2medium Russet potatoes, diced

Dash Italian seasoning

Salt & pepper to taste

Scallions chopped, optional

Preparation:

1. Cook bacon pieces in a large pot until crispy. This should take about 10 minutes. Set cooked bacon aside.

2. Add the chopped celery and onion to the pot and let it cook for 5 minutes. Add the flour, stir and cook for a minute or so.

3. Now add the garlic and pour in the stock; stir to dissolve flour and mix well. Add the chicken, the corn, the heavy cream, Italian seasoning, and 3/4 of the bacon. Cook on high heat and bring the soup to a boil.

4. Lower heat and simmer for 15 to 20 minutes, with frequent stirring, until the potatoes are done.

5. Add salt and pepper to taste and serve, garnished with the reserved bacon and scallion.

Nutrition Per Serving: *Calories: 548kcal | Fat: 26g | Carbs: 54g | Protein: 27g |Fiber: 4g| Cholesterol: 117mg| Sodium: 845mg*

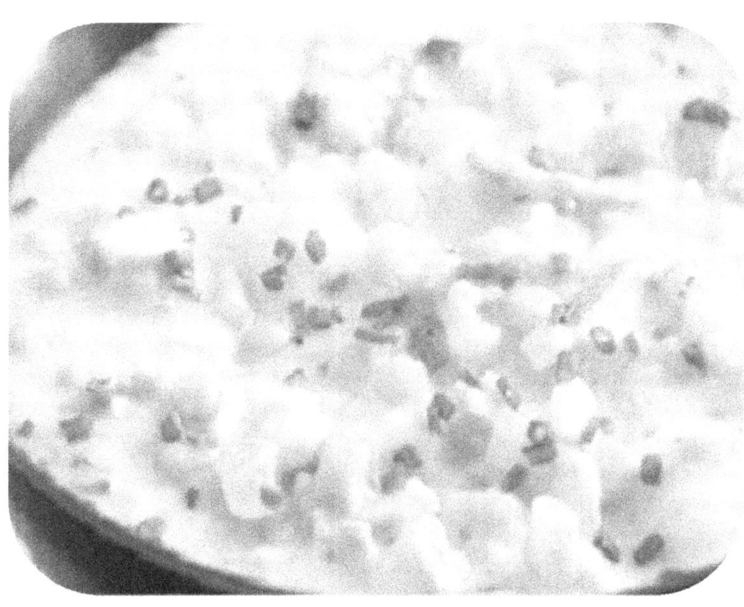

Stuffed Pepper Soup

A tomato-based hearty broth that includes ground beef, onions and peppers.

Prep Time 10 minutes

Cook Time 30 minutes

Servings: 6

Diet Phase: Solid food

Ingredients

1 tablespoon extra-virgin olive oil

1 pound lean ground beef

3/4 cup of chopped onion

1 1/2 teaspoons of minced garlic

Salt and pepper to taste

1 green bell pepper, cut into pieces

1 red bell pepper, cut into pieces

1 14.5 ounce small can of diced tomatoes

1 14.5 ounce can beef broth

1 15 ounce can tomato sauce

2 teaspoons of Italian seasoning

2 cups of cooked white rice

2 tablespoons of chopped parsley

Preparation:

1. Add the olive oil to a large pot and heat over medium high heat. Once hot, add the ground beef and cook for 5 minutes, breaking up into smaller pieces, until browned.

2. Add the onion and cook until softened. This should take 5 minutes or less. Add the garlic and cook for several seconds. Season with salt and pepper.

3. Now add the chopped bell peppers and cook for a few minutes. Add the tomatoes, the tomato sauce, broth and Italian seasoning and bring soup to a simmer.

4. Cook for 15 to 20 minutes and once the peppers are softened, add the rice in, stir and add more salt and pepper, as desired.

5. Serve, sprinkled with parsley.

Nutrition Per Serving: *Calories: 286kcal | Fat: 10g | Carbs: 28g | Protein: 20g |Fiber:3g| Cholesterol: 49mg| Sodium:769mg*

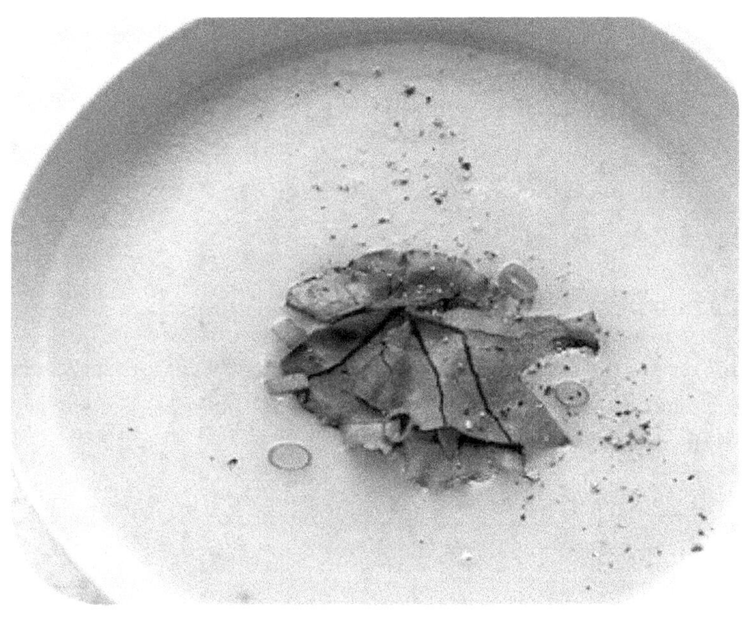

Potato leek soup

Potato Leek Soup

Prep: 10 minutes

Cook: 40 minutes

Servings: 4

Diet Phase: Pureed

<u>Ingredients</u>

4 cups chicken stock

4 russet potatoes

2 small leeks (whites only)

1 stalks celery

1 bay leaf

3/4 teaspoons of chopped fresh thyme

Salt and fresh ground pepper

½ cup heavy cream

<u>Preparation</u>:

1. Prepare the ingredients: peel the potatoes and cut into large pieces. Wash the white parts of the leeks and slice. Chop the celery roughly and chop the fresh thyme finely.

2. In a large pot, add the stock, potatoes, the leeks, celery, the bay leaf and thyme and season with salt and pepper, boil for 20 minutes until the potatoes are tender.

3. Discard the bay leaf. Blend soup with an immersion blender smooth. Add the cream and simmer about 20 minutes to thicken.

Nutrition Per Serving*: Calories: 245kcal | Fat: 12g | Carbs: 32g | Protein: 6g |Fiber:5g| Cholesterol: 40mg| Sodium: 1436mg*

Creamy Chicken Cauliflower Soup

A healthy, low carb, gluten free and dairy free comforting soup recipe.

Prep Time: 25minutes

Cook Time: 60minutes

Servings: 4

Diet Phase: Soft food

Ingredients:

1 lb. chicken breast boneless, skinless

1 cauliflower head, cut into florets

1 cup unsweetened coconut milk or milk of choice

4 cups of low sodium chicken broth

1 tablespoon of olive oil

2 teaspoon parsley

Salt and pepper

Preparation:

1. Preheat your oven to 350F. Place the chicken on a paper-lined baking sheet Sprinkle it with salt and pepper and drizzle with oil.

2. Bake the chicken for 30 minutes.

3. In the meantime, place the cauliflower florets on a large baking sheet evenly. Roast in the oven for 25 minutes or until tender. Remove and let it cool for 10 minutes.

4. Blend the cauliflower in a food processor. Add the milk and blend to smoothness. Now add the broth, parsley, the salt and the pepper and blend to smoothness until thick and creamy.

5. Place the mixture in a large pot, cover and bring to a boil on medium heat.

6. Shred the chicken with 2 forks and add to the pot.

Meal Prep:

1. Place in an airtight container and store in the refrigerator forup to 7 days or place in the freezer and store for up to 60 days.

2. When ready to eat, remove and heat for 10 minutes.

Nutrition Per Serving*: Calories: 346kcal | Fat: 21g | Carbs: 11g | Protein: 29g |Fiber: 4g| Cholesterol: 72mg| Sodium: 1656mg*

Ginger And Turmeric Chicken Soup

A highly nutritious, immune-boosting soup to keep you healthy!

Prep Time: 15 minutes

Cook Time: 50 minutes

Servings: 6

Diet Phase: Pureed

Ingredients

2 tablespoons olive oil

1 small onion, diced

3 celery stalks, diced

3 garlic cloves, minced

1 tablespoon fresh ginger, grated

2 medium sweet potatoes, (about 1 pound) skinned and cubed

2 lb. boneless, skinless chicken breast

5 cups chicken broth

1 teaspoon fresh thyme, chopped

1/2 teaspoon coarse sea salt

1/4 teaspoon black pepper

2 teaspoons turmeric

1 bay leaf

1 cup of coconut milk

1 head kale, (remove stem and chop roughly)

2 tablespoons lemon juice

<u>Preparation:</u>

1. In a pot, melt the butter. Add chicken to melted butter and cook on both sides until browned. This should take about 5 minutes.

2. Add the onion and add the celery as well and cook for about 5 minutes or a little more until tender. Add the garlic and the grated ginger and cook until fragrant or for a minute.

3. Place the chicken back to the pot. Add the sweet potatoes and pour in the chicken broth, add the seasoning: salt, pepper, thyme, turmeric and bay leaf. Place the lid on and cook 40 minutes on medium heat or until chicken is very tender and can be pulled apart easily with a fork.

4. Remove chicken, shred with two forks. Return to pot, add the coconut milk, stir and add the kale. Cook until kale is wilted. This should take 2-3 minutes.

6. Add the lemon juice and adjust seasonings as needed. Spoon into bowls

Nutrition Per Serving: *Calories: 402kcal | Fat: 16.9g | Carbs: 23.5g | Protein: 40g |Fiber:3.7g| Cholesterol: 110.3mg| Sodium: 336.7mg*

Seafood Tofu Stew

Prep Time: 15 minutes

Cook Time: 50 minutes

Servings: 2

Diet Phase: soft food

Ingredients

1 and 1/2 cup mixed seafood

Salt and pepper

1 teaspoon cornstarch

2 teaspoons canola oil

1 teaspoon ginger, sliced

2 tablespoons green onion, chopped

1 lb. soft tofu, cubed

1 cup mushroom

2 cups chicken stock

Preparation:

1. Use a paper towel to pat dry the mixed seafood and place in a bowl. Sprinkle with a little salt and pepper. Mix and then add the cornstarch, mixing thoroughly. Let it rest for 10 minutes to marinate.

2. Meanwhile, add the oil to a pan and heat and then add the ginger and the green onion. Stir and cook and then add the seafood. Stir and cook for a minute. Turn off heat.

3. Spread the tofu in a Dutch oven. Place the seafood and vegetables on the tofu in the oven. Add the chicken broth and let it boil for medium heat. Lower heat, cover and simmer for 10 minutes. Season with salt and pepper. Serve warm.

Nutrition Per Serving*: Calories: 207kcal | Fat: 8.2g | Carbs: 9.2.g | Protein: 25g |Fiber:1.8g| Cholesterol: 109mg| Sodium: 545mg*

Pureed Broccoli Soup

Prep Time: 10minutes

Cook Time: 15minutes

Servings: 4

Diet Phase: Pureed food

Ingredients

1 tablespoon butter

1 tablespoon olive oil

1 medium onion, chopped

2 cloves garlic, chopped

1 stalk celery, chopped

1 teaspoon fresh thyme, chopped

8 cups broccoli, chopped

2 cups water

4 cups reduced-sodium chicken or vegetable broth,

½ teaspoon salt

Preparation:

1. Add butter to pot and when it melts, add the oil and then add the onion and the celery to the hot oil. Cook and stir for 5 minutes and then add the garlic and the thyme. Cook and stir for 10 seconds until fragrant.

2. Add the broccoli and then pour in the water and broth. Let it simmer over high heat and then place the heat on low and let it simmer for about 10 minutes.

3. Puree the soup until smooth. Use an immersion blender or use a blender and puree carefully in batches. Season with salt and pepper.

4. ***Make ahead:*** refrigerate, covered for up to 4 days. Freeze for up to 3 months.

Nutrition Per Serving*: Calories: 160kcal | Fat: 2.8g | Carbs: 16.5g | Protein: 8.7g |Fiber:5.4g| Cholesterol: 434mg| Sodium: 699mg*

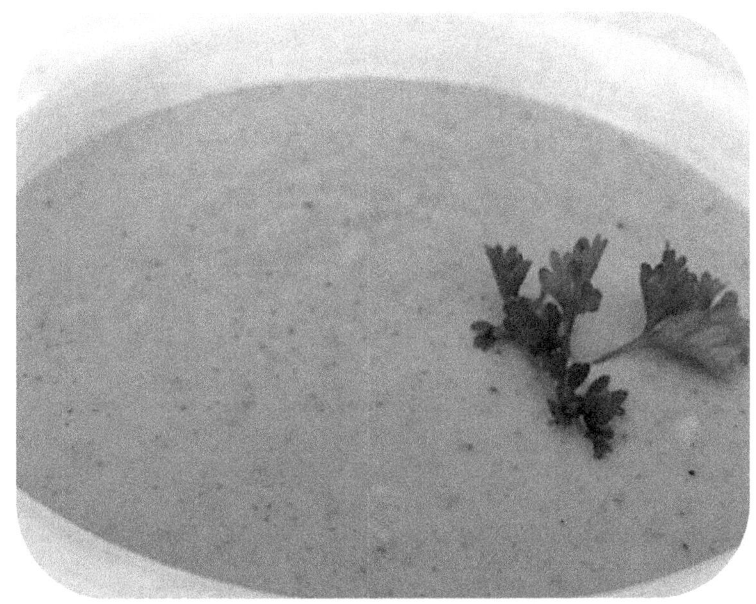

Taco Soup

Prep Time: 5minutes

Cook Time: 6 hours

Servings: 8

Diet Phase: Soft food

Ingredients

2 lb. ground beef

1-1/2 cups of water

1 tablespoon of taco seasoning

1 (15- oz.)can black beans, drained

1 (16- oz.) can mild chili beans, un-drained

1 (10-oz.) can diced tomatoes with green chilies

1 (15-1/4 oz.) can whole kernel corn, drained

1 (14 1/2- oz.) can of stewed tomatoes

2 1/2 tablespoons of ranch seasoning mix

1 (4- oz.) can chopped green chilies, optional

Preparation:

1. Brown ground beef in a pan for 5 minutes. Drain the excess fat.

2. Place in the slow cooker and then pour in the water. Add the rest of the ingredients. Stir to combine thoroughly.

3. Cook for 6 hours on low. Serve, garnished as desired.

Make ahead:

1. Store the soup in an airtight container and refrigerate for up to 3 days.

2. To store in the freezer, cool soup and place in a freezer-safe container for up to 3 months.

Nutrition Per Serving: *Calories: 390kcal | Fat: 23g | Carbs: 19g | Protein: 25g |Fiber:4g| Cholesterol: 81mg| Sodium: 707mg*

Veggie Pesto Soup

Prep Time: 5minutes

Cook Time: 35minutes

Servings: 4

Diet Phase: Solid food

Ingredients

1 tablespoon extra-virgin olive oil

2 medium cloves garlic, peeled & smashed

4 spring onions, (white and green parts), sliced thinly

2 medium carrots, peeled and thickly sliced

2 stalks celery, peeled and thickly sliced

2 leeks, (white and green parts), peeled and thickly sliced in half-moons

1 bulb fennel, cored & sliced

Kosher salt

6 cups of vegetable stock

1 bay leaf

1/2 cup peas

1 zucchini, peeled into ribbons

Freshly ground black pepper

1 1/2 tablespoons pesto

<u>Preparation:</u>

1. Cook garlic in heated oil for about 2 minutes, remove and discard.

2. Add the spring onions, the carrots, leeks, fennel and celery, add salt cook and stir for 5 minutes.

3. Pour in the stock, add the bay leaf and bring to boil. Simmer and cook about 15 minutes. Add the peas and zucchini, stir and simmer for a minute. Remove from heat.

4. Add the pesto, stir and sprinkle with salt and pepper. Discard bay leaf

5. ***Make ahead:*** cool and refrigerate for up to 3 days. To reheat, microwave for 2 minutes

Nutrition Per Serving: *Calories: 152kcal | Fat: 9g | Carbs: 14g | Protein: 4g |Fiber:6g| Cholesterol: 2mg| Sodium: 449mg*

Brazilian Shrimp Soup

Prep Time: 10 minutes

Cook Time: 20minutes

Servings: 4

Diet Phase: Soft food

<u>Ingredients</u>

1 tablespoon of olive oil

1 small onion chopped

½ of red bell pepper chopped

2 garlic cloves minced

¼ cup of rice long-grain

Dash red pepper flakes

½ teaspoon salt

14. oz. crushed tomatoes

2 cups of water

1/2 cup unsweetened coconut milk

9 oz. medium shrimp, shelled and cut

Pinch black pepper ground

11/2 tablespoons of lemon juice

¼ cup of fresh parsley, chopped

<u>Preparation:</u>

1. Heat the oil in a large pot and then add the onion, chopped bell pepper, and the minced garlic and cook for 5 minutes, with occasional stirring until tender.

2. Now add the rice, pepper flakes, tomatoes, salt and water and let it boil. Cook the rice for 10 minutes until done.

3. Add the coconut milk, stir and let it simmer, add the shrimp, stir and simmer for about 5 minutes until the shrimp is done.

4. Add the black pepper, the juice of lemon and the parsley.

5.***Make ahead:*** Store in an airtight container, refrigerated for up to 4 days.

Nutrition Per Serving: *Calories: 216kcal | Fat: 5g | Carbs: 21g | Protein: 11g |Fiber:2g| Cholesterol: 71mg| Sodium: 757mg*

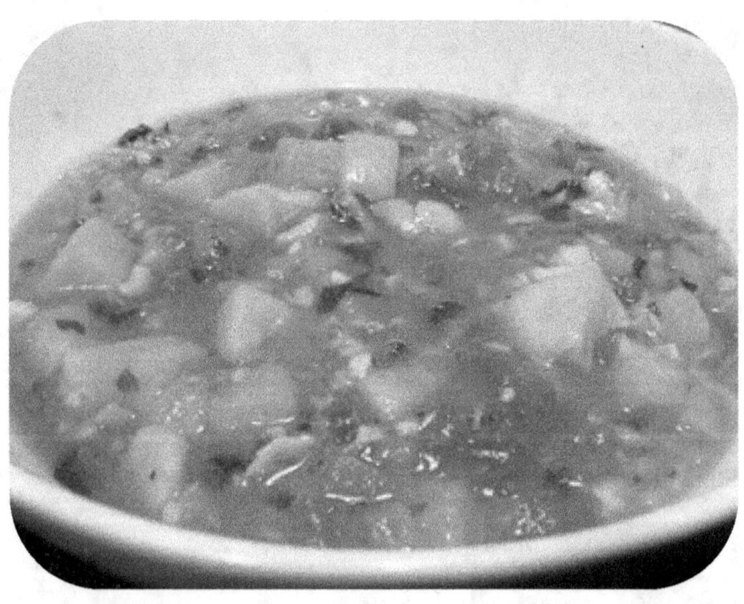

Fish Stock

Prep Time: 10 minutes

Cook Time: 20minutes

Servings: 8 1/2 cups

Diet Phase: Clear Liquid

Ingredients

2 pounds cod, sea bass bones or meaty halibut,

1 large onion, thinly sliced

1 large leek, (white and green parts), thinly sliced

1 sprig flat-leaf parsley

1 bay leaf

1 sprig thyme

3 peppercorns

Preparation:

1. Rinse the fish bones and place in a pot. Add the rest of the ingredients and pour 10 cups water as well. Bring almost to a boil. Lower heat and cook for 30 minutes. Skim any foam that rise to the surface.

2. Line a fine-mesh sieve with cheesecloth and strain the stock through it onto a pot or measuring cup. Discard solids.

3. *Make ahead:* cool stock, place in the refrigerator without covering and once cold. Remove, transfer to an airtight container and place in the freezer for up to 2 months.

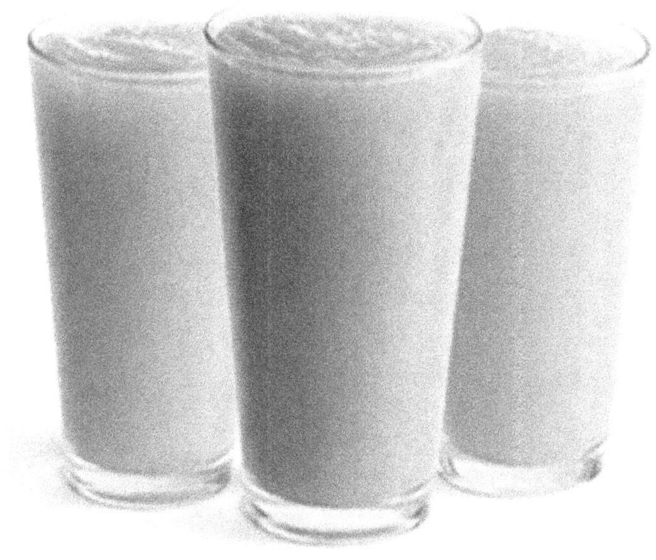

Blueberry Avocado Protein Smoothie

Prep/Total Time: 5 minutes

Servings: 1

Diet Phase: Full Liquid

Ingredients

1/2 medium avocado

1 cup frozen blueberries

1 cup of unsweetened almond milk

1/3 cup of egg whites

1 small scoop of stevia extract

1 scoop of vanilla protein powder

Preparation:

1. Blend all the ingredients in a Vitamix blender. Serve!

Nutrition Per Serving: *Calories: 388kcal | Fat: 14.3g | Carbs: 29.3g | Protein: 35.4g | Fiber:13.2g | Cholesterol: 5mg | Sodium: 350mg*

Kale Greens Smoothie

Prep/Total Time: 5 minutes

Servings: 2

Diet Phase: Pureed

Ingredients:

Medium handful kale

Medium handful spinach

1 inch of ginger, peeled

1/2 of a cucumber

1/2 cup broccoli

1/4 avocado

1/2 cup broccoli

1/4 cup of parsley

1/2 pear

1 lemon, juiced

Pinch of cayenne pepper

Warm green tea

Preparation:

1. Dice the broccoli, ginger, cucumber and avocado. Chop the pear.

2. Add all the ingredients, the tea inclusive, into a blender and blend until smooth.

3. Transfer to a cup and serve.

Nutrition Per Serving: *Calories: 150kcal | Fat: 3g | Carbs: 22g | Protein: 8g |Fiber: 4g| Cholesterol: 0mg| Sodium: 11mg*

Chocolate Banana Oat Smoothie

Prep/Total Time: 5 minutes

Servings: 1

Diet Phase: Pureed

Ingredients

¼ cup of oats

½ cup of oat milk

½ medium fresh banana

½ cup of coconut yogurt

1 ½ tablespoons of almond butter

2 scoops of chocolate protein powder

Preparation:

1. Add all the ingredients into the blender and blend mixture in short bursts.

Nutrition Per Serving: *Calories: 284kcal | Fat: 13g | Carbs: 28g | Protein: 17g |Fiber: 2g| Cholesterol: 60mg| Sodium: 170mg*

Mango Smoothie

Prep& Total Time: 3minutes

Servings: 2

Diet Phase: Pureed

<u>Ingredients:</u>

1/2 cup of yogurt

2 cups of frozen mango

1/2 cup of dairy-free milk

Chunks of 1 medium banana

<u>Preparation:</u>

1. Combine all ingredients to a blender and pulse it until the mixture is smooth and creamy.

Nutrition Per Serving*: Calories: 329kcal | Fat: 8.6g | Carbs: 64g | Protein: 6.3g |Fiber: 7.2g| Sodium: 27.7mg*

Yogurt& Chia Smoothie

Creamy, delicious and satisfying!

Prep& Total Time: 3minutes

Servings: 1

Diet Phase: Full Liquid

<u>Ingredients:</u>

2 tablespoons of full fat Greek yogurt

½ cup fresh strawberries

1 tablespoon chia seeds

1 cup nut milk

2 tablespoons of whey protein powder

Preparation:

Blend all ingredients until smooth.

Nutrition Per Serving: *Calories: 216kcal | Fat: 12g | Carbs: 15g | Protein: 15g |Fiber: 7g| Sodium: 41mg|Cholesterol 28mg*

Veggie Fruit Smoothies

In one glass, you have your daily nutritional requirements!

Prep& Total Time: 5minutes

Servings: 3

Diet Phase: Pureed

Ingredients:

2 cups of coconut water

1 cup of spinach

1 cup of watercress

4 celery stalks

2 carrots

1 clove garlic

1 red bell pepper

1 large tomato

1 red jalapeno, seeded, optional

Preparation:

1. Process all the ingredients in a food processor or blender.

Nutrition Per Serving: *Calories: 73kcal | Fat: 0g | Carbs: 14g | Protein: 1g |Fiber: 3g| Sodium: 138mg|Cholesterol 0mg*

Strawberry Orange Ginger Smoothie

Prep& Total Time: 5minutes

Servings: 2

Diet Phase: Full Liquid

Ingredients

1¼ cups of orange juice

1 banana

1 (1 inch) cube of fresh ginger root, peeled

2 cups frozen strawberries

Preparation:

1. Peel the ginger root and add to a blender together with the rest of the ingredients. Blend until smooth.

Nutrition Per Serving: *Calories: 185kcal | Fat: 1g | Carbs: 45g | Protein: 3g |Fiber: 5g| Sodium: 5mg|Cholesterol 0mg*

Bell Pepper Smoothie

Prep& Total Time: 5minutes

Servings: 4

Ingredients

1medium banana, peeled fresh or frozen

1 can (8 oz.) pineapple, drained

1/2 cup of red bell pepper

2 cups of frozen mixed berries

1 cup of water

Preparation:

1. Peel the banana. Deseed the red bell pepper and chop.

2. Combine all ingredients in a food processor and blend. Serve!

Nutrition Per Serving: *Calories: 100kcal | Fat: 0g | Carbs: 25g | Protein: 1g |Fiber: 8.3g| Sodium: 0mg|Cholesterol 0mg*

Almond Butter Berry Smoothie

Serves: 1

Ingredients

1/2 medium ripe banana

1/4 cup low-fat milk

1 tablespoon of creamy almond butter

1 cup raspberries, fresh or frozen

1/2 cup crushed ice

Preparation:

Blend and enjoy!

Pineapple Green Smoothie

Packed with vitamins and minerals, this super-healthy smoothie is worth every sip!

Prep& Total Time: 5minutes

Servings: 2

Diet Phase: Full Liquid

Ingredients

1 cup of preferred non-dairy milk

1 frozen banana

1 cup of baby spinach

1 cup of pineapple chunks

Preparation:

Blend all together in a high-speed blender. Enjoy!

Nutrition Facts: *Per Serving; Calories 131; Fat 2g; Carbohydrates 28g; Protein 1g; Fiber 6g; Sodium:13mg;*

Apple Carrot Kale Smoothie

Prep& Total Time: 5minutes

Servings: 2

Diet Phase: Full Liquid

Ingredients

1 cup of matcha green tea

1 cup of kale

1/2 cup carrots, skin on

1/2 large apple, skin on

1 frozen banana, peeled

3/4 cup of ice

1 whole date

1 tablespoon of chia seed

Preparation:

1. Add ingredients to a high powered blender, with the frozen banana last.

2. Blend for 11/2 minutes or thereabout. Enjoy!

Nutrition Facts*: Per Serving; Calories 161; Fat 2g; Carbohydrates 35g; Protein 4g; Fiber 7g;Sodium: 38mg; Cholesterol: 0 mg*

Creamy Carrot Orange Smoothie with Turmeric& Ginger

An immune boosting smoothie that's so creamy, and delicious!

Prep Time: 10 minutes

Cook Time: 1 minute

Servings: 2

Diet Phase: Pureed

Ingredients

8 baby carrots

1 teaspoon of water

1 orange, peeled

3 tablespoons of vanilla protein powder

1/3 cup Greek yogurt

1/2 frozen banana

1/4 teaspoon of ground turmeric

1/2 teaspoon of grated fresh ginger

1 teaspoon of honey

8 ice cubes

Preparation:

1. Place the baby carrots in a bowl. Add the water, cover and cook a minute on high heat. Remove once soft.

2. Place the cooked carrot in a blender and add the orange, protein powder, Greek yoghurt, banana, the ginger and the turmeric to it. Process for 2

minutes or process until smooth. Scrape the sides of the blender where necessary.

3. Add the honey and the ice cubes and blend until evenly mixed. Serve immediately.

Nutrition Facts: *Per Serving; Calories 132; Fat 0g; Carbohydrates 20g; Protein 4g; Fiber 3g; Sodium: 56mg; Cholesterol: 0 mg*

Wild Berry Mango Kefir Smoothie
A gluten-free, dairy-free, Paleo, vegan and vegetarian anti-inflammatory delight.

Prep& Total Time: 5minutes

Servings: 2

Diet Phase: Full Liquid

Ingredients

1-16 ounce Mango coconut kefir (Kevita brand)

2 cups wild blueberries, frozen

1 ripe banana, peeled &halved

½ teaspoon pure vanilla extract

¼ teaspoon of Ceylon cinnamon

1 tablespoon chia seeds

Organic stevia, to taste

2 cups baby spinach

Preparation:

1. Blend all the ingredients in a high speed blender until smooth and creamy.

Nutrition Per Serving: *Calories: 269kcal | Fat: 3g | Carbs: 54g | Protein: 8g |Fiber: 11g| Sodium: 53mg|Cholesterol 5mg*

Berry, Watermelon& Ginger Smoothie

Prep/Total Time: 10 minutes

Diet Phase: Pureed

Servings: 2

Ingredients

1 heaping cup watermelon chunks

1½ cups mixed berries, frozen

1 inch piece ginger, peeled &chopped or grated

2 teaspoons chia seeds

¾ cup coconut water

¼ Hass avocado

Preparation:

Blend all the ingredients and serve.

Nutrition Per Serving: *Calories: 180kcal | Fat: 5g | Carbs: 33g | Protein: 3g |Fiber: 5g| Sodium:2mg|Cholesterol 38mg*

Ginger Berry Mix

Prep/Total Time: 10minutes

Diet Phase: Pureed

Servings: 2

<u>Ingredients:</u>

2 inch piece of peeled ginger

1 cup of mixed frozen berries (cranberries, strawberries blueberries)

3 tablespoon of Nutiva hemp protein powder

2 cups of leafy greens (collards, kale, chard, romaine or spinach)

1 cup celery

1/2 cup water

<u>Preparation:</u>

1. Place all the ingredients in a blender and blend until smooth. Enjoy!

Nutrition Per Serving*: Calories: 94kcal | Fat: 2g | Carbs: 17g | Protein: 8g |Fiber: 7g| Sodium: 55mg|Cholesterol 0mg*

153

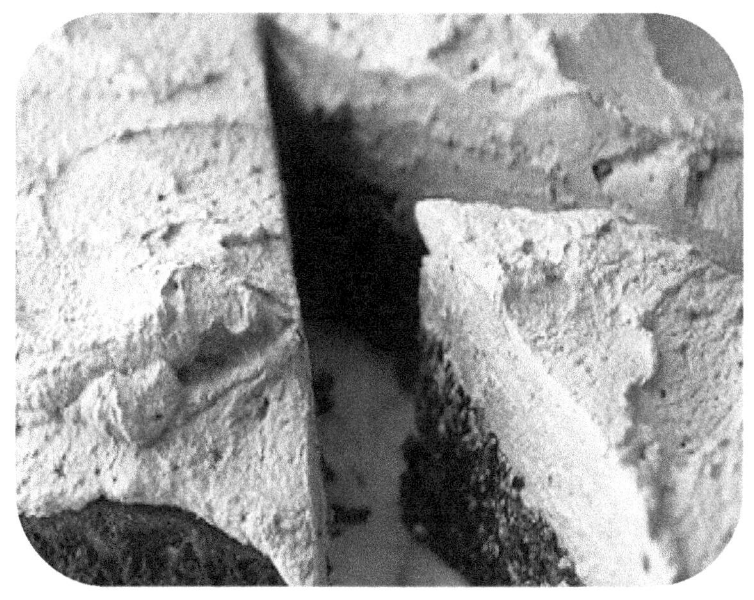

Banana Peanut Butter Ice Cream

Prep Time: 2 hours

Total Time: 2 hours

Servings: 4

Diet Phase: Soft food

Ingredients:

4 large ripe bananas

2 tablespoons peanut butter

Preparation:

1. Peel bananas, slice into discs and freeze 2 hours on a large plate.

2. Process until smooth. Add the peanut butter and process as well. Add 2 tablespoons of milk, if desired, for a more creamy consistency.

3. *Make Ahead:* freeze or refrigerate for up to a week.

Nutrition Per Serving Calories: 152kcal | Fat: 4g | Carbs: 29g | Protein: 3g| Fiber4g | Sodium: 38mg |

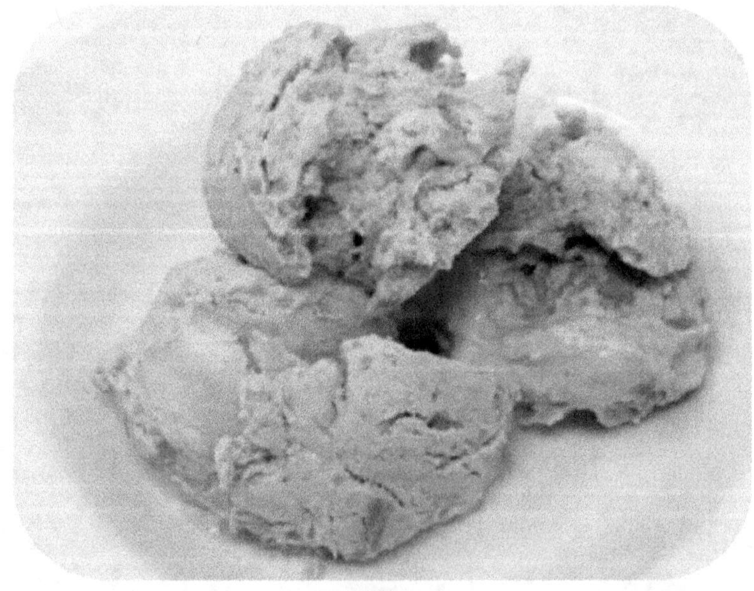

High Protein Vanilla Pudding

Prep Time: 2 minutes

Total Time: 2 minutes

Servings: 1

Ingredients

3/4 cup of Greek yogurt

1 scoop of vanilla powder (brown rice protein)

1-11/2 tablespoons of coconut flour

Preparation:

1. Add yogurt to a bowl. Add the protein powder and mix to fully incorporate.

2. Add the flour, mix well to desired consistency.

3. Refrigerate to thickenfor up to a week or enjoy immediately.

Nutrition Per Serving*: w/o toppings; Calories 180; Fat 1g; Carbs 14g; Protein 31g;*

Frozen Fruity Pops
Refreshingly cool Mango, Kiwi & Raspberry frozen pops!

Prep Time: 15 minutes

Cook Time: 5minutes

Servings: 4

Diet Phase: Solid food

Ingredients:

9 tablespoons of water

2 tablespoons of sugar, optional

5 oz. kiwi, peeled

6 oz. mango, peeled

6 oz. fresh raspberries

Preparation:

1. In a small pot, add together the water and sugar and let it boil on medium heat for 5 minutes. This is the syrup.

2. Add the fruits to a high-speed blender and puree. Pour into 3 small bowls.

3. Divide the syrup between the bowls of fruit purees, mixing in.

4. Transfer to 4 small cups and freeze for an hour. Add the mango puree and freeze for 20 minutes. Place sticks in and freeze 3 hours. Finally, add raspberry puree and 8 hours or freeze overnight.

5. ***Make ahead:*** freeze for up to 3 months.

Nutrition Per Serving (per pop) *Calories: 91.5 kcal | Fat: 0.5g | Carbs: 22g | Protein: 1g | Fiber4g | Sodium: 1.8mg |*

Chocolate Chip Cookie Dough (Whole Wheat)

Prep/Total Time: 10minutes

Servings: 2

Diet Phase: Stabilization

Ingredients:

3 tablespoons of stevia

1 tablespoon of brown sugar

2 tablespoons of softened butter

5 tablespoons of whole wheat white flour

1/8 teaspoon of vanilla

1/8 teaspoon of salt

2 tablespoons of dark chocolate chips

1/2 tablespoon of fat- free milk

Preparation:

1. Cream the sweetener, brown sugar and butter together. Stir in the flour, vanilla salt, and milk. Add the chocolate chips, to incorporate. Enjoy!

2. ***Make ahead:*** refrigerate for up to 2 days.

Nutrition Per Serving *Calories: 228kcal | Fat: 10.8g |Carbs: 35.4g | Protein: 2.8g| Fiber3.7g|Sodium: 239.3mg |*

Pumpkin Pie

Low carb and just perfect!

Prep Time: 10 minutes

Chill Time: 50 minutes

Servings: 8

Diet Phase: Soft food

Ingredients:

Pie Crust:

1 cup of almond flour

2 tablespoons of powdered swerve

1/4 cup coconut oil,

Filling:

3 eggs

1/2 cup heavy whipping cream

2/3 cup powdered swerve

11/2 teaspoons pumpkin pie spice

15 oz. canned pumpkin puree

1 teaspoon vanilla extract

Topping:

1/2 cup heavy whipping cream

Preparation:

1. Preheat the oven to 350F.

2. Combine the almond flour and sweetener in a bowl. Pour the melted coconut in it and mix until crumbly.

3. Transfer to a shallow pie pan, patting evenly into the bottom with your fingers. Prick the bottom of the crust with a fork.

4. For the filling, whisk together the eggs, cream, sweetener, pumpkin pie spice, canned pumpkin purée and pour into the pie crust.

5. Bake in preheated oven for 50 minutes. Cover the sides of the crust with foil.

6. Let it cool completely and then refrigerate.

7. ***Make ahead:*** refrigerate for at least 8 hours before slicing. This helps it to set well.

Nutrition Per Serving *Calories: 285kcal | Fat: 27g |Carbs: 9g | Protein: 6g| Fiber3 |*

Bitter Chocolate Mousse

With a higher cacao percentage, this chocolate mousse delivers a slightly bitter flavor that makes this dessert unique!

Prep Time: 20minutes

Chill Time: 2 hours

Servings: 6

Diet Phase: Solid food

Ingredients:

¾ cup of chilled heavy cream

4 large egg yolks

¼ cup of room temperature strong coffee or brewed espresso

1/3 teaspoon kosher salt

3 tablespoons sugar

6 oz. semisweet chocolate, chopped

2 large egg whites

Preparation:

1. Beat ½ cup of cream in a small bowl; cover and place in the refrigerator.

2. In a heatproof bowl, add together the egg yolks, coffee or espresso, salt and 2 tablespoon of sugar. Set over a saucepan of simmering water but ensure bowl does not touch the water. Whisk until the color is lighter and mixture is twice its volume. This should take about a minute.

3. Remove bowl from heat. Add the chocolate and whisk until smooth. Continue to whisk from time to time, until it is room temperature.

4. In a medium bowl, beat egg white with an electric mixer until foamy. Beat in the 1 tablespoon of sugar that's left. Raise the speed and beat until stiff peaks form.

5. Now fold the egg whites into the chocolate mixture; adding twice. Fold the rest of the whipped cream into the mixture, blending well. Transfer the mousse to 6 teacups and refrigerate for at least 2 hours until firm.

6. To serve, whisk remaining cream (1/4 cup) into small bowl and top each mousse cup with a dollop.

7. **Make ahead:** cover and refrigerate mousse for up to 1 day. To serve, remove and cool for at least 10 minutes.

Nutrition Per Serving *Calories: 290kcal | Fat: 22g | Carbs: 24g | Protein: 20g | Fiber 2g | Sodium: 85mg | Cholesterol 175mg*

Lemon cupcakes

Lemon Cupcakes

Prep Time: 20 minutes

Chill Time: 20 minutes

Servings: 12

Diet Phase: Solid food

Ingredients:

Cupcakes:

1/2 cup of softened unsalted butter

3/4 cup granulated sugar

2 large, room temperature eggs

1 tablespoon lemon zest

1 teaspoon vanilla extract

1/4 cup fresh lemon juice

1/4 cup whole milk

1 1/2 cups flour

1 1/2 teaspoons baking powder

1/4 teaspoon of salt

3/4 cup lemon curd

Frosting:

1 cup softened unsalted butter

1/8 teaspoon salt

3 1/2 cups of confectioners' sugar

4 tablespoons of fresh lemon juice

1 tablespoon lemon zest

Preparation:

1. For the cupcakes, first preheat your oven to 350°F and then place liners in 12 muffin cups; set aside.

2. Combine the butter and sugar and beat for about 5 minutes until fluffy. Add the eggs, one after the other; mix and add the lemon zest and vanilla, beating well.

3. Combine the milk and lemon juice in a measuring cup with a spout and set aside.

4. In a bowl, add together the flour, the salt and baking powder, whisk and then transfer to the butter mix and then to the milk mixture alternately. Beat thoroughly after adding.

5. Transfer the batter to the 12 lined muffin cups and bake for 20 minutes. Let it cool for 10 minutes. Take cupcakes out from pan and cool fully on a wire rack.

6. Once cupcakes are thoroughly cooled, cut the centre and fill with a tablespoon of lemon curd and frost it.

7. To make the frosting, beat the butter to smoothness. Use an electric hand mixer. Add the salt and beat to incorporate. Add a cup of confectioner's sugar, beat on medium –low speed and when the sugar is humidified, beat the lemon zest in and add the remaining sugar, little by little. Beat until all the sugar is humidified.

8. Add 2 tablespoons of lemon juice and beat on high speed until fluffy.

9. ***Make ahead:*** cover and store the cupcakes at room temperature for up to 1 day. Store the frosting in an airtight container and refrigerate for up to 1 day. Store frosted cupcakes air-tightly in a container and refrigerate for up to 3 days. Freeze cupcakes; either frosted or unfrosted, for up to 3 months. Place in the refrigerator overnight to thaw.

Nutrition Per Serving *Calories: 102kcal | Fat: 3g | Carbs: 18g | Protein: 3g | Fiber1 | Sodium: 135mg | Cholesterol 35mg*

Date Sweetened Chocolate Quinoa Cake

A gluten free, sugar free chocolate dessert.

Prep Time: 10minutes

Chill Time: 20minutes

Servings: 8 large slices

Diet Phase: Soft food

<u>Ingredients:</u>

1/2 cup raw quinoa, cooked to 1 1/2 cups quinoa

1 cup of dates

1/3 cup of coconut oil

2 eggs

1 teaspoon vanilla

1/4 cup cocoa powder

1/4 cup arrowroot powder

1/2 teaspoon salt

1/2 teaspoon baking soda

<u>Preparation:</u>

1. Preheat oven to 350F.

2. Pit dates, pour boiling water over it and let it rest to soften for a minute or two. Drain dates, add to a food processor, together with the cooked1 1/2 cups quinoa. Process to break up dates for 1 or 2 minutes.

3. Add coconut oil, the eggs, and the vanilla, and process an additional 1 to 2 minutes. Batter shouldn't be completely smooth, though.

4. Add the cocoa powder, arrowroot powder, salt and baking soda. Pulseand stir with a spoon.

5. Pour into a paper-lined baking pan, smooth the top with a spoon and bake for 30 minutes. Cool 15 minutes and cut into bars.

6. *Make ahead:* store in the refrigerator for up to 4 days. Freeze in an airtight container for up to 3 months.

Nutrition Per Serving *Calories: 213kcal | Fat: 10g | Carbs: 30g | Protein: 3g | Fiber 3g | Sodium: 205mg | Cholesterol 36mg*

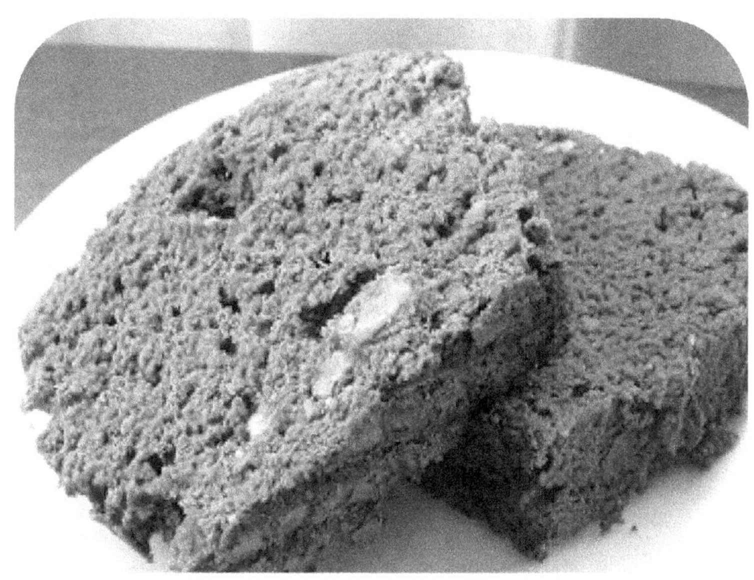

Lemon Berry Muffins

Muffins with finely ground strips of lemon zest? Now why wouldn't it have a sparkling flavor!

Prep Time: 10minutes

Chill Time: minutes

Servings: 12

Diet Phase:Soft food

Ingredients:

Zest of 1 lemon

½ cup sugar

1 cup nonfat buttermilk

1/3 cup canola oil

1 teaspoon vanilla extract

1 large egg

1 cup white whole-wheat flour

1 cup all-purpose flour

1 teaspoon baking soda

2 teaspoons baking powder

¼ teaspoon salt

1½ cups fresh raspberries

Preparation:

1. Preheat oven to 400F. Spritz 12 large muffin cups with non-stick cooking spray.

2. Add lemon zest and sugar to a food processor and pulse to chop contents finely. Add the buttermilk, the oil, vanilla and egg. Pulse to blend.

3. In a large bowl, add together the all-purpose flour,whole-wheat flour,baking soda, baking powder, and salt. Fold in the buttermilk mixture to almost blend and then add the raspberries, folding in.

4. Divide into prepared muffin cups and bake for 25 minutes or until the tops and edges are golden. Cool for 5 minutes in pan and then remove to cool on a wire rack.

5. *Make ahead:* wrap each muffin cup in plastic and place in a freezer bag to freeze for up to 1 month. To reheat, remove plastic, wrap the muffin in a paper towel and place in the microwave for 30 to 60 seconds.

Nutrition Per Serving *Calories: 182kcal | Fat: 6.8g | Carbs: 27g | Protein: 3.9g | Fiber2.4g | Sodium: 259mg | Cholesterol 16mg*

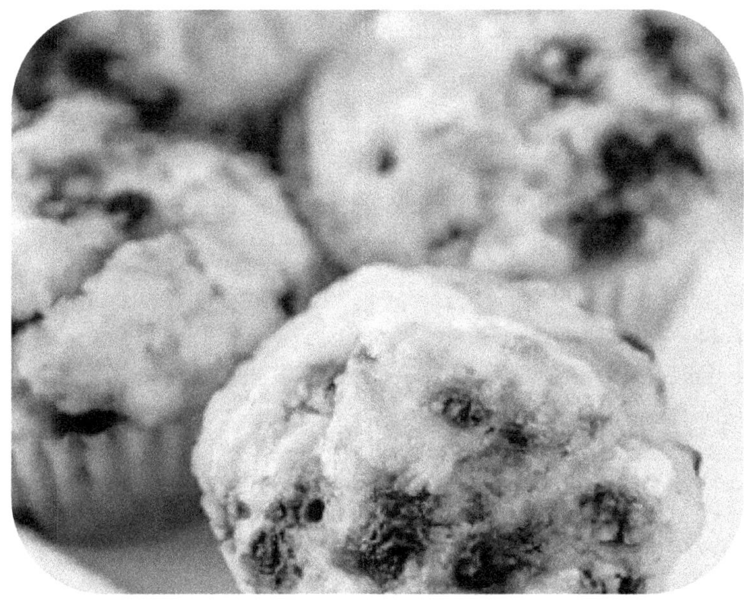

Cherry Chip Ice Cream

A delightful vegan make-ahead dessert!

Prep Time: 10minutes

Total Time: 3 hours 10minutes

Servings: 3 servings of ½ cup

Diet Phase: Soft food

<u>Ingredients:</u>

2 cups of fresh cherries

1/2 banana

1/2 cup of unsweetened almond milk

3 tablespoons of no-dairy chocolate chips

<u>Preparation:</u>

1. Wash the cherries, dry and remove pits. Freeze in a freezer bag for at least 3 hours.

2. Place ½ of a peeled banana in the freezer.

3, Pour 1/4 cup of the unsweetened almond milk into ice cube trays. Freeze the remaining ¼ cup of almond milk for at least 3 hours.

4. Transfer the frozen cherries, frozen half banana, the almond-milk ice cubes, and 1/4 cup of almond milk to a food processor. Process for 3-5 minutes until thoroughly smooth. Add the chocolate chips, stir, and eat immediately.

5. ***Make-ahead:*** ingredients can be frozen for up to 3 days before using.

Nutrition Per Serving *Calories: 126kcal | Fat: 4g |Carbs: 22.3g | Protein: 2.1g| Fiber2.8g|Sodium: 39mg | Cholesterol 2mg*

Concluded!